Shōnishin

of related interest

Baby Shiatsu
Gentle Touch to Help your Baby Thrive
Karin Kalbantner-Wernicke and Tina Haase
Foreword by Dr. Steffen Fischer
Illustrated by Monika Werneke
Translated by Anne Oppenheimer
ISBN 978 1 84819 104 4
eISBN 978 0 85701 086 5

Children at Their Best
Understanding and Using the Five Elements to Develop
Children's Full Potential for Parents, Teachers, and Therapists
Karin Kalbantner-Wernicke and Bettye Jo Wray-Fears
Translated by Anne Oppenheimer
ISBN 978 1 84819 118 1
eISBN 978 0 85701 093 3

Qigong Massage for Your Child with Autism
A Home Program from Chinese Medicine
Louisa Silva
Foreword by Dr. Anita Cignolini
ISBN 978 1 84819 070 2
eISBN 978 0 85701 041 4

Yoga Therapy for Every Special Child
Meeting Needs in a Natural Setting
Nancy Williams
Illustrated by Leslie White
ISBN 978 1 84819 027 6
eISBN 978 0 85701 027 8

Shōnishin

The Art of Non-Invasive Paediatric Acupuncture

Thomas Wernicke
With a contribution by Professor Wolfgang Michel
Translated by Anne Oppenheimer

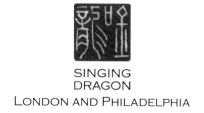

SINGING
DRAGON
LONDON AND PHILADELPHIA

First published in 2014
by Singing Dragon
an imprint of Jessica Kingsley Publishers
73 Collier Street
London N1 9BE, UK
and
400 Market Street, Suite 400
Philadelphia, PA 19106, USA

www.singingdragon.com

Library of Congress Cataloging in Publication Data
A CIP catalog record for this book is available from the Library of Congress

British Library Cataloguing in Publication Data
A CIP catalogue record for this book is available from the British Library

ISBN 978 1 84819 160 0
eISBN 978 0 85701 117 6

Printed and bound in China

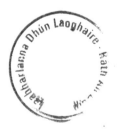

Contents

Acknowledgements

My heartfelt thanks go first and foremost to the countless babies and children who had such trust in me and let me treat and learn from them. In their company there were sunny moments that lit up my life.

Thanks also to my 'back family', which gives me a home and makes my back strong. To my partner in practice, my wife Karin, with whom, over almost 30 years of shared interest, I have devoted myself to investigating child development in the East–West context. She has shown me again and again how important it is to have a vision; without it I would soon have come to a halt. To my daughter Yana, whose heart and skill as a photographer are so wonderfully evident in this book.

I am so thankful to my revered teacher Tanioka-sensei in Ōsaka, who opened wide for me the gate into the child's world. His very special way of treating with Shōnishin struck a chord with me that has proved a key influence in my professional development.

I'd like to express my very special thanks to Professor Michel for his expert support. I was able to raise his interest in exploring the historical background of paediatrics in ancient Japan. This he did with a great deal of hard work and enthusiasm, and in so doing has made an important contribution, not only to this book in particular, but also to the cultural history of Japan in general. Thanks to his work on the original literature of the Edo and Meiji periods, Shōnishin can now be evaluated as a paediatric treatment.

From history back to the present: here I would like to express my sincere thanks to the parents of the wonderful 'models' for giving permission to photograph their children. And, last but not least, a heartfelt 'thank you' to my publisher, Jessica Kingsley. She didn't know what she was letting herself in for when taking on this book, but with no knowledge of Shōnishin she trusted in me the first time we spoke and, with no 'ifs and buts', agreed to the project straightaway.

Preliminary Notes on Treating Children

Children aren't small or unfinished grown-ups. Children live in the world of their own thoughts and feelings, with their own potential and abilities – which we, as adults, have often lost, or at any rate forgotten about. Nevertheless, as grown-ups we think that we are cleverer or more able than children. But when you are in contact with children, this attitude seems presumptuous. Depending on the circumstances they have experienced or suffered, children have a far more comprehensive and profound – and in part more onerous – experience than adults. As adults 'working' with children, this is something we should always be aware of.

There is a noticeable trend among therapists of attaching increased importance to the treatment of babies and children. This development springs from the recognition, first, that children are the most precious thing their parents have; and second, that timely intervention in case of disorders or abnormalities can save much pain and therapy later in life.

So many professional groups have 'discovered' the child for themselves. This is to be welcomed. But unfortunately it can be seen, among the various groups of professionals, that treatments offered for children are on the increase in spite of inadequate or even non-existent knowledge of the specific characteristics of children. So the following questions arise: What needs special attention when treating children? And what is special about them?

To begin with, it's important to be aware that in agreeing to treat children, one is taking on a great responsibility. This is true also for the Shōnishin acupuncturist. It's all the easier to understand if we take a closer look at the following circumstances leading up to treatment with Shōnishin.

While many babies are easy to care for, others may have particular requirements. If the baby cries often and is difficult to soothe, mother or father faces a big challenge, especially if the baby is their first child. If the parents then bring their child to a Shōnishin acupuncturist, it is usually with less high expectations or hopes. Often, uncertainty, or even fear, plays an important part for parents. Ultimately they are, as a rule, bringing their child for Shōnishin because they are worried. Many have not always been taken seriously by paediatricians, so feel alone with their worries, uncertainties and unanswered questions:

- Something is the matter with my child!

- Why?

- Why is she crying all the time?

- Why can't she walk yet?

- Why doesn't she want to play with the other children at playgroup?

- Why does she always have a headache at, or after, school?

- Why does she find some things more difficult than other children do?

- Why is she often left out by other children?

In the end they seek help from their midwife, the educational advisory service or the special 'crying unit', buy self-help books and are lectured by their in-laws about their parenting style.

What we are looking at here is the classic young parent scenario – confusion guaranteed! Because everything they hear or have read about in books looks rather different in practice, beginning with mother-and-baby groups, where children of the same age are crawling – or not – and each one is different. Every single child is at a different point of development. In a situation like this it's inevitable that parents will compare their own baby with others.

'Anna can crawl already and my Matty can't yet – is everything OK with my child?' And that is precisely the question the Shōnishin acupuncturist is asked when he is treating Matty.

In situations like this, parents need four things:

1. certainty

2. trust

3. clarity

4. essential knowledge about the stages of child development.

A Shōnishin acupuncturist can only provide these if he knows what he is doing. If, for example, he isn't familiar with child development, then he will struggle in a situation like the one described above. This knowledge is essential.

Thus, a child cannot be treated without the help of the parent or caregiver. This is especially true with babies. Therefore, a Shōnishin acupuncturist should also be able to offer expert support to the parents within the treatment context; for example, by:

- demonstrating what is physiologically the best way of lifting, carrying and handling a baby

- providing expert advice on the right way for a baby to lie in her cot

- not least, answering questions on important developmental stages.

When treating children – and this is especially the case with babies – time plays an important role. The younger a child is, the faster she reacts to treatment, regardless of whether it's an osteopathic, homoeopathic or Shōnishin treatment. This, as a rule, makes treating children (especially babies) easier than treating adults.

It is important to be mindful that the optimum timescale within which a child can be treated varies, depending on age. The younger a child is, the shorter the timescale for optimal treatment. This means, for example, that treating a crooked baby with KISS Syndrome (Kinetic Imbalances due to Suboccipital Strain) at the age of 6 weeks or 6 months – whatever the therapy – will make an enormous difference.

For the Shōnishin acupuncturist this means that in some circumstances another therapeutic intervention is necessary in addition to Shōnishin, to avoid letting an opportunity pass. But it can also mean that a different therapy should be introduced in good time because the child is not responding to Shōnishin. This is a question of recognising one's own limits, and the limits of whatever the other therapy might be, besides the corresponding reaction to treatment.

Finally, as my revered Shōnishin teacher Tanioka-Sensei puts it, in Shōnishin there is a single goal: to give children back their laughter. To which I would add: …and the parents too.

Part I

Theoretical Principles

1

Historical Background
Treating Children in Japan

Professor Wolfgang Michel

1.1 Lost traditions

There is no lack of discussion in Japan today on the subject of children, childhood and youth. Many problems, some serious, arose from the second half of the nineteenth century, in a turbulent change of course following the fall of the Tokugawa Dynasty, as the country turned towards Western science and techniques, and in the course of only a few decades joined the first rank of industrial nations. The promoted separation between 'Japanese spirit and Western technology' (*wakon-yōsai*) was not as straightforward as had been envisaged, and Japan is still struggling to find its own identity and place in the world.

This also applies in the educational sphere. Stringent selection in schools inflicts wounds, and alongside all the problems of behaviourally disturbed children and young people there is the self-image of many educators, constructed as it is on the foundation of rigid discipline. Attempts at reform, which have been ongoing for decades, are failing to have the anticipated impact. Hardly surprising, then, that not only in education but also in the world of 'traditional' arts and sports, there are still niches where a rude, commanding tone and physical pressure are taken for granted.

However, this is by no means the legacy of time-honoured tradition. François Caron (1600–1673), who arrived in Japan as a cabin boy at the beginning of the seventeenth century and made a career for himself in the Dutch trade station of Hirado, and became thoroughly acquainted with the language, country and people, offered the following in reply to a question from the Director of the East India Company in Batavia:

Children are carefully and tenderly brought up; their parents strike them seldom or never, and though they cry whole nights together, endeavour to still them with patience; judging that infants have no understanding, but that it grows with them as they grow in years, and therefore to be encouraged with indulgence and examples.

It is remarkable to see how orderly and how modestly little children of seven or eight years old behave themselves, their discourse and answers savouring of riper age, and far surpassing any I have yet seen of their times in our Country.[1]

Similar observations can be found in other Western writings of the Edo period, whenever the authors cast a glance at childhood and education in the Empire of Nippon. After the country opened up in the nineteenth century this care and consideration persisted for a while, as we can see from the following description of a street scene by two scientists whom the Japanese government had sent into the countryside on a tour of duty:

The little ones' main playground is the street, where they pursue their games totally without concern for the traffic. They know that the pedestrian, the Jinrikisha-coolie with his vehicle, the carrier with his heavy burden, will not object to a small detour to avoid treading on the spinning top, upsetting the flight of the shuttlecocks in a game of *Hago-ita*, or interfering with the string of a kite; they see the horse approaching at a fast trot, and carry on playing, undisturbed. They are accustomed to being treated with respect.[2]

There are many reasons for the breakdown of this tradition. One thing that played an important role in education was the appointment of Emil Hausknecht (1853–1927), a disciple of German Professor Johann Friedrich Herbart (1776–1841), to the Chair of Pedagogy at the University of Tokyo. But the rising modern nation state was already making deep incursions into people's lives, and before long they were merged into a new 'national body'.

1.2 Children as a treasure

Children were a treasure, childlessness a misfortune. Many divinities took care of the blessing of children, of pregnant women, and the protection of children – first among them the bodhisattva Jizō (Ksitigarbha) (guardian of children) and the merciful Koyasu-Kannon (giver of children and easy delivery).

From pregnancy and birth until death, life was accompanied by rituals.[3] A few have survived to the present day. For example, the umbilical cord is kept as an amulet. For a while after delivery, young mothers move back to their parents' homes with their infants (the period of seclusion). The first visit with the infant to a Shintō shrine is still important to many families. In addition, there are seasonal festivals with Chinese roots, such as the doll festival on the third day of the third month, and the boys' festival on the fifth day of the fifth month.

Customs that were once practised predominantly by the Samurai class became unified in the Meiji era into the form of a countrywide 'Seven-Five-Three Festival' (15 November). On this day parents take their 3-, 5- and 7-year-old children, magnificently dressed, to the shrine to give thanks for the years so far and ask for protection for a long life to come.

With the introduction of compulsory schooling the traditional children's groups in the areas around the shrines have disappeared. All-day school attendance and all manner of after-school tuition mean that little time is left for socialisation within the family. Now, starting and finishing elementary school, junior high school and senior high school are important ceremonial events for the entire family.

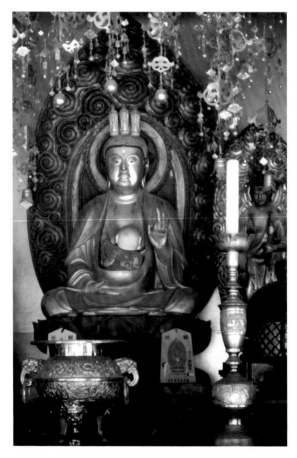

Figure 1.1: Koyasu-Kannon (Enryū-Temple, Nakatsu, Oita Prefecture)
For followers of Christianity, which was forbidden during the Edo era, statues like this were substitutes for figures of the Virgin Mary.

1.3 Children as a burden

The history of childhood in Japan also has a dark chapter on the abortion of foetuses ('water children'), infanticide of unwanted newborns and exposure of children. In some cases, such as the birth of twins, there were 'cultural' reasons for this. But for the most part it was sheer destitution that drove families to 'weeding out' (*mabiki*).[4] Failed harvests, earthquakes, fires or excessive tax burdens imposed by the territorial rulers led to repeated famines and uprisings among the rural population.

The feudal lords, in fear of agricultural decline in their domains, tried to restrict these infanticides by means of prohibition. However, there was no fundamental improvement until after the Meiji Restoration (1868), when the first institutions for foundlings and orphans were formed. At the same time laws were introduced by several stages to make abortion, and sale of the means to carry it out, punishable offences. The new citizen had become a valuable unit of labour, all the more so when an expansion of the national territory became imminent.

1.4 Education

Traditionally, education played an important role,[5] regarding which Caron has the following to say:

> None go to school under seven or eight years of age, as being until then incapable of its rules, and more inclined to play than to learn, unless it be waggishness and wantonness. At school they begin by degrees, by sweetness and not by force, the masters imprinting an ambition and desire in each of them to out-go his fellow; they lead them likewise by example, telling them that such and such learned so much in so little time, whereby his honour and family was so highly advanced. The children are so accustomed to this way that they learn sooner and more than by any correction or whipping; for generous spirits and an obstinate nation, such as this is, are not to be forced, but rather won with gentleness and emulation.[6]

Antoine François Prévost (1697–1763) also established that the Japanese would neglect nothing 'that could improve the minds of their children', and 'in this respect [they made] no distinction between the sexes'.[7]

In China almost every office in the imperial administration was open to aspirants of all classes through examinations that were held countrywide. The Japanese bureaucracy of the early modern period, on the other hand, originated in the class of the Samurai, who served their feudal lords as sword-bearing officials once peace had been established in the archipelago. In comparison with

Chinese 'civil servants', their attitude showed more aggressive traits and a strong bond with the feudal lord in any given case.

For a long time the character of the Japanese empire was shaped by Buddhism. Buddhist monks, as cultural ambassadors, brought many things into the country from their travels in China, including Chinese medicine and other scientific achievements. From the fourteenth century onwards, with the adoption of new Chinese techniques in silk weaving, metallurgy and shipbuilding, craftsmen and merchants acquired a more powerful influence on technical and scientific thinking. The struggles over hegemony in the fifteenth and sixteenth centuries, connection into the European global network and the rise of Japanese long-distance trade created the conditions for increasing social and intellectual flexibility.

This was not altogether in the interests of the Tokugawa, who had gained control of the country at the beginning of the seventeenth century. To consolidate their rule ideologically, they promoted the teachings of the Chinese Neo-Confucian Zhuxi (*Shushi* in Japanese, 1130–1200). He had developed a vast system that embraced the individual, society and the universe and forced human relationships into a hierarchical straitjacket. Alongside respect and righteousness, industriousness and ambition were established virtues.

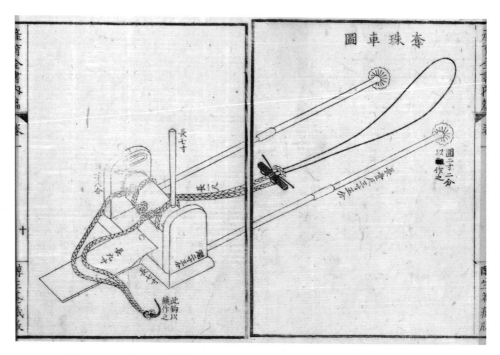

Figure 1.2: Forceps (dakyūsha) used in obstetrics (Mizuhara Yoshihiro: Saniku zensho, 1850. Courtesy Ken-i-kai Library, Tōkyō)

In the Japan of the early modern period we can see a considerable increase in the number of educational institutions.[8] Besides the traditional Buddhist temple schools and feudal schools for the children of the Samurai, large numbers of private schools came into being. Many were focused on the Chinese classics, while others espoused the so-called 'Dutch Studies' (*rangaku*). In addition, there were countrywide circles that pursued all kinds of arts, and also strict disciplines like mathematics, for pleasure.

Notwithstanding the complexity of the writing system, the standard of literacy skills was higher than in Europe. The output of the printing trade in the Edo era, in the traditional form of wood block printing, ranged from manuals, dictionaries and encyclopaedias, via literary texts of all kinds, to practical texts such as nobility directories, cookery books, travel guides and advice on how to bring up children.[9]

1.5 Paediatrics as an independent branch of medicine

Paediatrics was established as an independent branch of medicine in the early days of the Japanese Empire. The state institutions of the Nara era (710–784) were built on a modified Chinese foundation. In health care there was elaborate medical legislation which regulated physicians' training, legal status and professional activity. For the 'main path' (which roughly corresponds to present-day internal medicine) there was nine years' training, for surgery seven years, and for treating conditions of the eyes, ears, mouth and jaw (as well as for 'magical practices'), three years in each case. Paediatrics, with five years' training, was in third place. Graduates from these courses looked after the aristocracy, at court and in the regions. Treating the common people was left to the Buddhist temples, or anyone who felt they had the vocation for it.

The first general synopsis of medicine in Japan, the *Ishinhō* (or *Ishimpō*) by Tamba Yasuyori, contains chapters with titles such as 'Women', 'Obstetrics' and 'Children'. For a long time Chinese teaching was adopted more or less unaltered. Not until the twilight of the Middle Ages was there any shift away from this. One of the pioneers of this emancipation, Manase Dōsan (1507–1594), wrote the first germane book in Japanese, *Prescriptions for Longevity in Children* (*Karei shōnihō*) in 1568. More works, like the *Marvellous Home Remedies* (*Kachinhō*, 1577) by Itasaka Sōkei, followed. Many of these are dedicated to the child in the family (*ie* in Japanese, *ka* in Sino-Japanese) and include, besides the treatment and prevention of disease, all sorts of questions on how to bring up children. The handbooks on childrearing that were printed in large numbers during the Edo era were also written mainly by physicians, who interpolated chapters on health care and home remedies.[10] Occasionally, physicians from China came to Nagasaki on Chinese merchant ships and brought new medical knowledge into the country. In this way Zhōu Qílái, who landed in Japan in 1725, was responsible for disseminating the *Diverse Views on Paediatrics* (*Yòukē shézhōng*) by Qín Chāngyùe.[11]

In the seventeenth and eighteenth centuries, Japanese medicine became further detached from Chinese models. In aetiology as well as therapeutic interventions, Japanese innovations began to appear, with increased emphasis on observation and experience. Some physicians dedicated themselves exclusively to paediatrics. At the court of Hidetada (1579–1632), the second Shōgun of the Tokugawa dynasty, one paediatrician was considered sufficient, but under his successor Iemitsu (1604–1651) there were seven. In 1691, the German physician Engelbert Kaempfer registered two paediatricians (*shōnigata*) of Shōgun Tsunayoshi (1646–1709).

With a reorganisation of the health care system during the Ming dynasty in China, traditional massage (*ànmó*, 'pressing and rubbing') was re-named in 1571. Soon afterwards Gōng Yúnlín used the new term (*tuīná*, 'pressing and grasping') in his book on child massage, *Secret Principles of Child Massage* (*Xiǎoér tuīná mìzhǐ*, 1604). In Japan the old name, *anma*, persisted, but now encompassed new Japanese techniques as well. Relevant books of the later Edo era, such as the influential *Handbook of Anma* (*Anma tebiki*, 1800) or *Illustrated Abdominal Massage* (*Anpuku zukai*, 1827), also contain chapters on how to treat children.

A range of activities was performed, predominantly by visually impaired and blind people. There is the famous tradition of itinerant blind musicians and storytellers. After many years of arduous effort Sugiyama Wa'ichi (1610–1694), who became blind in childhood, opened up massage and acupuncture as a new profession for blind people, and even gained support for this from the Tokugawa government.[12] The school he founded in 1693 is recognised as the world's first educational institution specifically for the visually impaired. Some of the privileges that were granted at that time continued into the twentieth century.

At the same time, in the eighteenth century, Western medical literature began to be translated, and read not just by devotees of 'Dutch Studies' (*rangaku*). In the field of paediatrics the Japanese translation of *The Diseases of Children and their Remedies* by the Swedish author Nils Rosén von Rosenstein (1706–1773) was a pioneering achievement. The work reached Japan in the Dutch edition (*Handleiding tot de kennis en geneezing van de ziekten der kinderen*), which was published in 1779. There it was translated by the scholar Udagawa Genshin (1769–1834) and posthumously published in 1845 by his son Yōan.[13]

The fall of the Tokugawa dynasty and the birth of the Meiji government in 1868 brought radical changes. While traditional medicine was placed under severe restrictions, in 1870 it was decided to introduce Western standards in training and practice, following the principles of the German medical system. The first institutionalised department of paediatrics was created at the new University of Tokyo in 1888, when the doctor Hirota Tsukasa (1859–1928) returned from studying with Oswald Kohts (1844–1912) in Strasbourg. His *Paediatric Vademecum* (*Jika hikkei*, 1888) served medical students and practitioners as the new discipline's standard work. In 1895, following a course of study in Berlin, Itō Sukehiko became director of the children's clinic in Fukuoka. Some years later the clinic was incorporated into the clinic of the new Imperial University of Kyushu. In 1903 Hirai Ikutarō, on his return from Breslau (present-day Wroclaw), became head of the children's clinic at the Imperial University of Kyōto. 1895 saw the first appearance of the specialist journal *Shōnika* (*Paediatrics*), which the following year changed its title to *Jika zasshi* (*Acta paediatrica Japonica*). In 1903 it received, on the back page, a German title: *Zeitschrift für Kinderheilkunde und Schulhygiene* (*Journal of Paediatrics and School Hygiene*). In 1901 the Scientific Working Group on Paediatrics (*Shōnika kenkyūkai*), which had been established at the end of 1896, became the Paediatric Society (*Shōni kagakukai*). Up until World War I the principles of paediatric training and practice followed the Western style throughout the country.[14]

1.6 Childhood diseases in early modern books

For the Edo era (1603–1867), 13 large measles epidemics are recorded. In the last one, in 1862, around 240,000 people perished in Edo alone. No less feared was smallpox, which had ravaged the country approximately every 30 years from the eighth century onwards. For centuries, despite intensive studies, people were virtually helpless. At the end of the eighteenth century the practice of variolation, which had been introduced from China, became widespread in Kyushu. In the mid-nineteenth century Otto G. Mohnike (1814–1887) introduced vaccination, as developed by Edward Jenner.

Manase Dōsan explains in his *Remedies for Longevity in Children* that the bodies of children and adults are different. Most childhood diseases were caused, in his opinion, by 'womb poison' (*taidoku*). According to Chinese tradition this toxin, which was caused by depression, faulty nutrition and unrequited sexual desire, entered the child's body through the womb or during childbirth, causing carbuncles, boils, eczema, scabies, and more besides. A further frequent cause of illness, wrote Manase, was 'harm caused by food' (*shokushō*).

The *Valuable Notes on Acupuncture and Moxibustion* (*Shinkyū chōhōki*, 1719) published by Hongō Masatoyo affords an excellent synopsis of the diagnostics, therapy and disease patterns of his time. This work, held in high esteem right up until the twentieth century on account of its methodical structure, contains a section on paediatrics. According to Hongō, treating children had been considered difficult since ancient times. This is hardly surprising, since, for one thing, the paediatrician could not carry out an oral interview with the patient (*monshin*), which was one of the four pillars of diagnosis in Sino-Japanese tradition. That was why Manase and others called paediatrics the 'mute subject' (*a-ka*) or 'children-mute-subject' (*shōni-a-ka*). Hongō asserts, further, that the pulse is not yet fully established, which meant that another important diagnostic procedure could not be used. With children under the age of three, all that that could be done was to judge by the skin tone in parts of the face (forehead, lower jaw, chin and nasal region), and also the colour and pattern of the skin on the inside of the three phalanges of the index finger, flexed to meet the tip of the thumb in the position known as the 'jaws of the tiger' (*kokō sankan*). The Chinese doctor Yáng Jìzhōu had given a detailed description of this in his *Principles of Acupuncture and Moxibustion* (*Zhēnjiǔ dàchéng*). Hongō recommends a modified form of pulse diagnosis only for children over the age of 3.

On some sicknesses, he goes into a bit more detail. The 'wind of terror' illness (*kyōfū*; Chinese *jīngfēng*) accompanied by cramps and convulsions is probably a form of meningitis. The term that follows, *tenkan* (Chinese *diānxián*) is interpreted today as epilepsy. But for this condition in children Hongō uses different Japanese characters, and distinguishes – partly with regard to the 'five phases' (*gogyō*) – all kinds of different forms, using verbal prefixes with meanings like wind, sputum, food, drink, dogs, cattle, poultry, pigs and goats. In the case of the 'five storage organs' (five viscera, *gozō*) – the liver, heart, lungs, kidney and spleen – a differentiating condition called *kan* (Chinese *gān*) applies in all kinds of nervous phenomena, up to and including convulsions associated with abdominal pain, tension in the abdominal region, lack of appetite, skin discolouration and more. Further, he mentions intermittent fevers (*gyakushitsu, okori*), which can be treated together with jaundice (*ōdan*), and also constipation (*katakai*), vomiting and diarrhoea (*agekudashi, tosha*). This section concludes with a paragraph giving key-point summaries of problems in neonates.

Of course, decoctions, pills and powders were used for therapy. Hongō's work *Valuable Notes on Internal Medicine* (*Idō chōhōki*) gives a long list of these.[15] However, in almost every case he also applies needling or direct burning with moxa. Occasionally he draws small amounts of 'bad blood' (*oketsu*) from small blood vessels (*shiraku*).

Along with Chinese medicine the 'nine worms' that were held responsible for all kinds of illness arrived in Japan. Some of them were based on concrete observations of parasites. Others were theoretical constructs, and partly also had the rationale of making up the supposedly magical number nine. The illustrations were appropriately imaginative.[16]

The abdomen (*hara*) had a much more important role in the Japanese understanding of the body than it did in China. From antiquity it had been considered as the seat of the emotions and of thought, and many turns of phrase still bear witness to this today.[17] With increasing emancipation from Chinese medicine came new approaches, with the abdominal region as the locus of diagnosis and therapy. The number of worms (*mushi*) also increased significantly in Japan. Some of their names indicate the location where they lurk (ears, chest, lungs, intestine, spleen, kidney, etc.), and others the complaint they cause (abdominal pain, backache, fainting, etc.).

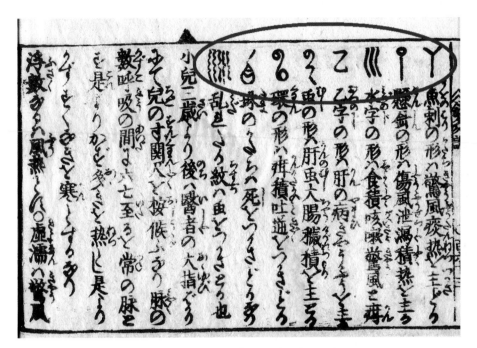

Figure 1.3: Pattern on the inside of the index finger (Hongō Masatoya: Shinkyū chōhōki, 1719. From the author's collection)

In the early modern period the worm concept was mixed in with other ideas on disease.

According to the dictionary of the Chinese Emperor Kāngxī (*Kāngxī Zìdiǎn*, 1716), the *kan* sickness in the 'five storage organs', mentioned above, was a result of excessive indulgence in sweet things (*kan*). Japanese paediatrics then added worms (*kan-no-mushi*) as a cause, and declared their extermination to be a treatment objective. For this, decoctions were used, and later on trade preparations such as the 'pill for the prevention of the five *kan* in children' (*Gokan-hodōen*) promoted by Ishida Teikan at the beginning of the eighteenth century. A shopping guide from the metropolis of Edo (*Edo kaimono hitori annai*) in 1894 lists six more preparations, among them the 'red toad pills' (*Reiden akahiki-gan*) that were traded by itinerant dealers up until the Meiji era. Some of the worms could be exterminated by means of acupuncture or moxibustion.

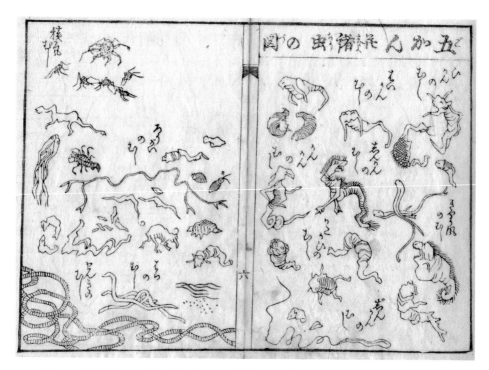

Figure 1.4: Worms of the five kan, and diverse other worms; below: a tapeworm (Ishida Teikan: Shōni yōiku kogane no ishizue, 1813. From the author's collection)

1.7 Non-invasive and mildly invasive procedures in the Sino-Japanese tradition

The history of Chinese acupuncture began with 'stone needles' (Chinese *biānshí*), which were used to make incisions in the skin or stimulate particular parts of the body. With the arrival of metal needles and the systematisation of medicine came the concept of the 'nine needles' described in *The Yellow Emperor's Inner Canon* (*Huangdi Neijing, Lingshu*). Some were used for puncturing, others as surgical lancets, and two types for acupressure and massage on the surface of the body: the round-tipped needle (Japanese *inshin/enshin*) and the blunt-tipped needle (Japanese *teishin*).

The Yellow Emperor's Inner Canon distinguishes nine different ways of needling (Chinese *jiǔbiàn*). In 'hair piercing' (Chinese *máocì*) the skin is pierced shallowly to treat superficial illness. At another place in the same book we find five further types of needling, with names linked to the five storage organs. In the first type of needling, 'half-needling' (Chinese *bàncì*), the needle is only superficially inserted and then immediately withdrawn, as if one were pulling out a hair. In this way the skin *qi* that corresponds with the lungs is supposed to be drawn out without injuring the skin.[18]

The Chinese needle types and needling techniques reached Japan, where, within the framework of new therapeutic concepts, more needles and (mostly invasive) techniques were developed. Renowned were the thick gold 'tapping needle' (*uchibari*) that was gently inserted with a little hammer, and the 'tube needle' (*kudabari*) that was inserted through a guide-tube. The former can be traced back to the monk Mubun and was further developed by Misono Isai (1557–1616); the latter was invented by Sugiyama Wa'ichi.

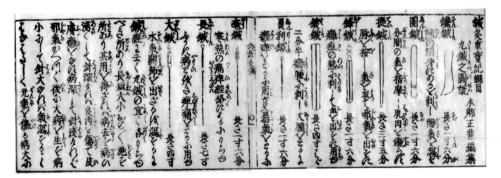

Figure 1.5: The classical 'nine needles' (Hongō Masatoyo: Shinkyū chōhōki, 1719. From the author's collection)

1.8 On the birth of paediatric acupuncture (Shōnishin)

Non- or mildly invasive procedures are part of the Chinese and Japanese medical traditions, but the paediatric acupuncture (Shōnishin or *shōnihari*: *shōni*, 'child'; *shin/hari*, 'needle, needling') of today was not the result of a long, historical course of development. It is in fact a young therapy that came into being in the early twentieth century in the region around Ōsaka.[19]

Up until well into the nineteenth century, invasive needling and direct moxibustion were by no means uncommon in the treatment of small children. Manase Dōsan, the pioneer of Japanese paediatrics, describes predominantly medicine-based therapies in his work *Karei shōnihō* (1568); later works also contain numerous remedies. But, as in Chinese medicine, acupuncture was widely used in Japan. This was done partly on traditional points (*tsubo*) along the meridians (*keiraku*, channels and tracts), and partly the meridians were ignored and places selected in the abdominal region and elsewhere.

In eighteenth-century Japan there was a renaissance of bloodletting from the smaller blood vessels (Japanese *shiraku*) using the 'three-edged needle' (as described in *The Yellow Emperor's Inner Canon*). European doctors at the trading station of Dejima, and the medically trained interpreter Yoshio Kōzaemon (1724–1800), had introduced Western-style venous bloodletting. Physicians of the Old School (*ko-ihō*) in particular, like Yamawaki Tōmon (1736–1782) and Ogino Gengai (1737–1806), saw this as confirmation of the classical Chinese precepts and attempted to bring Western and Japanese techniques into harmony.

Even the 'stone needle' (Japanese *henseki, ishibari* or *henseki*[20]) made its way into Japanese paediatrics,[21] after the influential Chinese doctor Xuē Kǎi and his son Xuē Jǐ (1486?–1558?) had recommended the use of sharp-edged porcelain shards for removing subcutaneous accumulations of 'cinnabar toxin' (*dāndú*, Japanese *tandoku*).[22] Moxibustion on children cannot have been pain-free, with three, five, even seven grains on the head, above the navel and on other sensitive spots[23] – to say nothing of surgical use of the 'three-edged needle' for all kinds of swellings, or for intestinal obstruction in newborn babies.

These procedures were used because they were considered indispensable. The risks were well known. In *The Yellow Emperor's Inner Canon* it says that small children have delicate flesh, little blood and weak *qi* (Japanese *ki*), therefore filiform needles (Chinese *háozhēn*) should be used, inserted shallowly and rapidly withdrawn.[24] And Hongō warns about using acupuncture or moxibustion on newborns without good reason. This might stir up the 'five storage organs' and set off illnesses.[25]

It was probably observed first in traditional massage (*anma*) that gentler approaches are not without effect in certain cases. The pioneering obstetricians Kagawa Genetsu (1700–1777) and his adopted son Genteki (1739–1779) introduced seven abdominal massage techniques (*anpuku*; *fuku/puku*, abdomen) for pregnant women.[26] Later writings on massage more or less consistently include a chapter on the subject, followed by a chapter on massage for infants. Ōta Shinsai, who systematised the techniques, wrote with reference to children that their organs are not yet developed and their skin, flesh, bones and tendons are still soft. As they are growing by both night and day, he said, they are affected by slight 'external evils' (*gaija*), as well as by the mother's milk and by food. Even healthy children should always be given abdominal massage. Then the milk and food will not cause blockages, elimination will be problem-free, the spirit strengthened and diseases prevented. Children hate medicine when they are ill. Abdominal massage, on the other hand, helps in most cases. Ōta gives a list of conditions for which experience had proved his therapy to be particularly effective: diarrhoea, bringing up milk, acute and chronic 'wind of terror' (*kyōfū*), besides 'cinnabar toxin' in skin conditions. As a child's abdomen is small, he limits his massage to two kinds. For pregnant women he recommends massaging the abdomen from the fourth or fifth month to regulate the position of the foetus and avoid miscarriage or premature birth.[27]

All these techniques and experience, however, did not necessarily lead to the birth of non-invasive acupuncture for children. Nagano Hitoshi, who was the first to examine the origin of Shōnishin therapy more closely, points out a significant external factor.[28] In 1885 a system of examination and certification had been introduced for acupuncturists and massage practitioners. In 1911 further restrictions were imposed on their field of activity. Following the Ministry of the Interior's announcement of new rules for controlling acupuncture and moxibustion practice, bloodletting (*shaketsu*), every kind of invasive surgical measure, electrical cauterisation and similar procedures, as well as the dispensing or prescription of medication, were prohibited. The rules came into force at the beginning of the following year.[29]

While in China traditional medicine was largely left in peace, in Japan doctors with a traditional orientation lost a large part of their therapeutic skillset. This existential crisis soon set off an intense quest for alternative methods, and for ways of saving and continuing to accumulate knowledge.

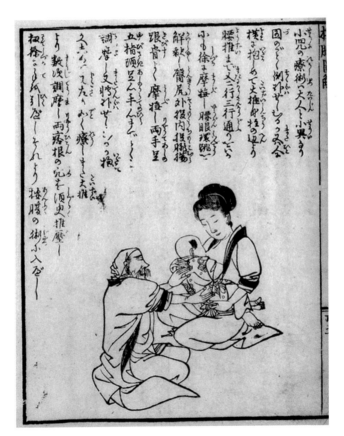

Figure 1.6: Infant massage (Ōta Shinsai: Anpuku zukai, 1827.
Courtesy of Kyushu University Medical Library)

1.9 Shōnishin pioneers

Many of the Japanese pioneers of the Edo era were high-ranking doctors. Sugiyama Wa'ichi was an official of the highest rank open to blind people. Yamawaki Tōmon rose to the second highest rank for a monk as a doctor. Ogino Gengai held high office as a physician at the court of Tennō in Kyōto. Ishizaka Sōtetsu (1770–1842), who sought to use Western anatomy for his acupuncture, held a no less prominent position at the court of the Shōgun in Edo. Thanks to their social status and lively publishing activity, their concepts are well documented. Non-invasive paediatric acupuncture, on the other hand, was done by town practitioners. Here, the need to prove therapeutic efficacy in everyday life took precedence over theoretical stringency, for these doctors had to secure 'market share' and earn a living. Successful new developments, therefore, were often passed on as 'secret tradition' only to sons and chosen disciples. For this reason the documentary evidence from the early phase of non-invasive acupuncture for children is very scarce.

In particular, acupuncturists in Ōsaka played an important part. Early nineteenth-century tables with rankings of local physicians give the names of several families (Nakano, Emura, Sugihara) specialising in acupuncture for children. They also show new needling techniques that were evidently established as 'brands': *Nakano hari* (Nakano needle), *Emura usagi hari* (Emura rabbit needle), *Sugihara usagi hari* (Sugihara rabbit needle). *A Directory of Physicians in Present-Day Ōsaka* (*Kinsei Naniwa ika meikan*), printed in 1845, also gives the name of Fujii[30] under acupuncture for children.

The Nakano family tree goes back to the ninth century. According to tradition it began with an encounter with Kūkai (774–835), also known as *Kōbō-daishi* (Grand Master Who Propagated the Doctrines). This outstanding thinker, after studying in China with the patriarch Huì Guǒ at the Blue Dragon Temple of Chang'an, brought esoteric Shingon-Buddhism to Japan. As in other Buddhist denominations, the monks of the Shingon Temples were also healers, who used the knowledge received from China for charitable ends. Even after Japanese medicine became more and more secularised towards the end of the Middle Ages, the memory of these Buddhist roots was cherished in many medical families. As an inscription on a map of the district around Hirano in the year 1763 (*Sesshū Hirano ōezu*) shows, the Nakano family was already specialising in acupuncture for children in the eighteenth century. During the Meiji era Nakano Shinkichi integrated elements of Western medicine into his practice. The nearby railway station and district of the city still bear the name of Hari-Nakano (*hari*, needle) today.

The physician and acupuncturist Takashima Bun'ichi, in his memoirs *The Way of the Needle – Youth of an Internist*, describes a non-invasive procedure that was practised in nearby Kyōto. For this, two connected pilot tubes were used. By gentle tapping of the first, empty tube, the needle in the second tube was made to vibrate and stimulate the selected point on the skin.[31]

The medical tradition of the Fujii family resident in Ōsaka began with Fujii Hidetaka, who published a text on *Illumination of Doubts in Acupuncture and Moxibustion* (*Shinkyū benwaku*, 1765). In addition to a chapter on problems before and after childbirth, the book contains some discussion of childhood diseases. Fujii Hidetaka explains that many childhood illnesses can be triggered by worms in the abdomen as a result of nutritional disorders. He consistently treated selected meridian points. Occasional claims that elements of a non-invasive technique could be found in this book have not been confirmed.

At the beginning of the twentieth century his descendant Fujii Hideji bridged the gap between traditional Japanese medicine and modern Western medicine, with his scientific studies of non-invasive paediatric acupuncture.[32] Takashima Bun'ichi kept up a close association with Fujii, who was 30 years his senior. According to Takashima, Fujii had studied with Professor Kasahara Michio (1883–1952) at the Imperial University of Ōsaka and in 1930, after experimenting with rabbits, had gained his doctorate with a thesis on non-invasive acupuncture for children. This was the first medical dissertation on acupuncture in Japan. Fujii kept all sorts of dogs and birds for his small patients in the garden of his practice. He used an ordinary steel needle with which he gently stimulated the points selected.[33] Fujii's studies made a significant contribution to recognition of the new therapy.

The Tanioka family had managed a small Shingon Temple since the Edo era. Presumably this got into financial difficulty after 1868, like many Buddhist temples in the aftermath of the Meiji reforms. Tanioka Sutezō (1857–1931) became blind at the age of five and, given the medical tradition of Shingon Buddhism, as well as the principles created by Sugiyama Wa'ichi in the seventeenth century, an obvious solution was for him to become a masseur or acupuncturist. There is no more exact information about the early years, but oral tradition has it that in 1876, a year after the new medical system came into force, he set up an acupuncture and moxa practice for adults and children. The fact that in 1888 he was granted a one-year training with the internist Yamaoka Miyoshi serves to emphasise the pressure the traditional healing professions were under at the time.

Tanioka used a three-edged needle with a rounded tip, which he drew backwards with a stroking motion over the selected point. This can be seen as the birth of acupuncture for children in the style of the 'Grand Master' (*Daishi-ryū Shōnishin*).[34] Tanioka Sutezō treated predominantly the area from the back of the head down to the shoulders and back. In the second generation, other parts of the body were included. As revealed by an information pamphlet that has come down to us, the attempt was made to combine the accumulated experience and insight acquired through practice, with scientific research. With reference to acupuncture, the above-mentioned Dr Fujii Hideji was the stated authority. For moxibustion, it was Hara Shimetarō (1882–1991). After graduating from the Prefectural Medical School in Kyōto, Hara completed a study on the effects of moxa on the immune system of rabbits with tuberculosis at the Imperial University of Kyūshū.[35] This was Japan's first medical dissertation on moxibustion, and Hara, who had been in practice since 1929 and later founded the Kashii Hara Hospital in Fukuoka, became famous across the country as the 'moxa doctor'. Tanioka Sutezō and his son Kentarō accumulated a wealth of knowledge, which has been shared with interested parties since the third generation. Thanks to the publications and lecturing activity of Tanioka Masanori, 'paediatric acupuncture in the manner of the Grand Master' (*Daishi-ryū Shōnishin*) is freely available today.[36]

By the beginning of the twentieth century, political and institutional pressure, together with revision (based on keen experimentation) of the achievements of traditional child massage and acupuncture, had led to the birth of a non-invasive paediatric acupuncture that linked conventional elements with new concepts, and bore remarkable results.

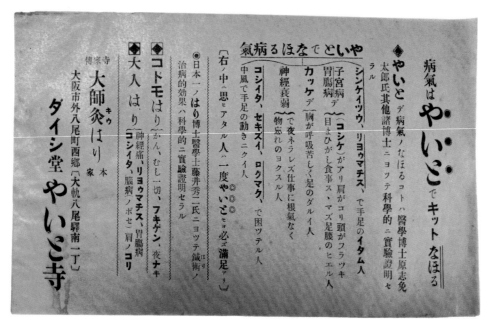

Figure 1.7: Daishi Temple leaflet from the 1930s giving information about the applications of moxibustion and acupuncture for adults and children, and making reference to Dr Fujii Hideji and Dr Hara Shimetarō (Courtesy of Tanioka Masanori, Ōsaka)

Notes

1   Caron (1663/1935), p. 48ff.
2   Netto/Wagener (1901).
3   For more on this, see Herold (1992)
4   For more, see Chiba/Ōtsu (1983) and LaFleur (1992)
5   More on this in Deal (2006)
6   Caron (1663/1935), p. 48ff.
7   Schwabe (1753), Book II, p. 597.
8   More on this in Dore (1965) and Deal (2006).
9   More on this in Kornicki (1998).
10 An outstanding example of this kind is Katsuki Gyūzan's *Handbook of Childcare and Childrearing* (1714).
11 Ōba (2003), pp. 186–189.
12 Kakinuma (1980), p. 8ff.
13 Udagawa (1845)
14 Shuku (1964), pp. 154–187.
15 Hongō (1733), p. 106ff.
16 c.f. *Gozō no shugo narabini mushi no zu.*
17 'read the inside of the abdomen' (read someone's mind), 'someone's mouth and abdomen are different' (he says one thing and means another), 'the abdomen is black' (conceal one's real intention), etc.
18 *Huángdì Nèijīng, Língshū*, Chapter 7 ('Guān zhēn').
19 The opinion of several authors that this tradition is several hundred years old has not been confirmed.
20 The Japanese name 'stone needle' appears for the first time in the dictionary *Setsuyōshū* (Kuromoto edition, fifteenth century) as *ishibari*.
21 Nagano (2010).
22 In the *Băoyīng cuōyào* the chapter 'Production of cinnabar toxin through womb poison' (*Tāidú fādān*, Vol. 11), in particular, gives a detailed description. Modern Japanese and Chinese medicine use the terms *tandoku* and *dāndú* respectively for erysipelas.
23 Hongō (1718), pp. 184–168.
24 *Huángdì Nèijīng, Língshū*, Chapter 38 ('Nìshùn féishòu').
25 Hongō (1718), p. 168.
26 Kagawa (1775), pp. 1–3.
27 Ōta (1827), pp. 75–77.
28 Nagano (2010), p. 409.
29 *Shinjutsu kyūjutsu torishimari kisoku*, Paragraph 7 (proclaimed on 14. August 1911, came into force on 1 January 1912).
30 Ozaki, Yamaguchi, Yoneyama (2012), p. 48ff.
31 Takashima (2004), p. 13ff.
32 Fujii (1927, 1929, 1940).
33 Takashima (2004), p. 14ff.
34 Wernicke (2009), pp. 1–3.
35 Hara (1929).
36 Tanioka (2005), Wernicke (2009).

Bibliography
Primary sources

Caron, F. *A True Description of the Mighty Kingdoms of Japan & Siam*. Reprinted from the English edition of 1663 with introduction, notes and appendixes by C.R. Boxer. Argonaut Press, London 1935

Chamberlain, B.H. *Things Japanese*. Kelly & Walsh, London 1905

Fujii Hidetake. *Shinkyū benwaku* [*Illumination of Doubts in Acupuncture and Moxibustion*]. [s.n.], [s.l.], [s.a.] (preface 1765)

Fujibayashi Ryōhaku. *Anma tebiki* [*Handbook of Anma*]. [s.n.], Edo 1800

Gōng Yúnlín. *Xiǎoér tuīná mìzhǐ* [*Secret Principles of Child Massage*]. [s.n.], [s.l.], 1604 (reprint: Tiānjīn Kēxué jìshù chūbǎnshè 2004)

Gozō no shugo narabini mushi no zu [*Protection of the Five Viscera and Illustrations of Worms*]. Manuscript, Edo-Period (Kyushu University, Medical Library)

Hirota Tsukasa. *Jika hikkei* [*Paediatrics*]. Kanehara Shoten, Tōkyō 1888

Hongō Masatoyo. *Idō chōhōki* [*Valuable Notes on Medicine*]. [s.n.], [s.l.], 1733 (preface 1709)

Hongō Masatoyo. *Shinkyū chōhōki* [*Valuable Notes on Acupuncture and Moxibustion*]. [s.n.], Edo/Ōsaka/Kyōto 1718

Huángdì Nèijīng, Língshū [*Yellow Emperor's Inner Canon, Spiritual Pivot*]. Táilián guófēng chūbǎnshè, Táiběi 1984 (sixth revised edition)

Imamura Ryōan. *Shinkyū shishō* [*Manual of Acupuncture and Moxibustion*]. Keigyōkan, Edo 1863

Ishida Teikan. *Shōni yōiku kogane no ishizue* [*Golden Foundation of Childrearing*]. [s.n.], Kyōto 1813 (revised editions 1851, 1865)

Itasaka Sōkei. *Kachinhō* [*Marvellous Home Remedies*]. [s.n.], [s.l.], 1577

Kagawa Genteki. *Sanron yoku* [Supplement to *The Theory of Obstetrics*]. Suharaya Mohē, Edo 1775

Katsuki Gyūzan. *Shōni hitsuyō sodategusa* [*Basic Handbook of Child Care*]. Kagaya Zenzō, Ōsaka 1714 (preface 1703)

Kinsei Naniwa ika meikan [*A Directory of Physicians in Present-Day Ōsaka*]. [s.n.], Ōsaka 1845 (reprint: Yamada Sakon (ed.). *Ika meikan zenhen – Kinsei Naniwa ika meikan kyōka 2 nen*. Ōsaka, Maeda Shoten 1970)

Manase Dōsan. *Karei shōnihō* [*Remedies for Longevity in Children*]. [s.n.], [s.l.], 1568

Mizuhara Yoshihiro. *Saniku zensho* [*Complete Book of Obstetrics*]. [s.n.], [s.l.], 1850

Nakagawa Gorōzaemon (ed.). *Edo kaimono hitori annai* [*Shopping Information for Edo*]. Yamashiroya Sahē, Edo 1824

Oka Ryōin. *Shōni imashimegusa* [*Instructions on Child Care*]. Chūkan sho'oku, [s.l.], 1820

Ōta Shinsai. *Anpuku zukai* [*Illustrated Explanations on Abdominal Massage*]. Okuda Yasuke, Ōsaka 1827

Qián Zhòngyáng (author), Yán Xiàozhōng (ed.), Xuē Jǐ (comm.). *Xiǎoér zhíjué* [*Secrets of Child Care*]. [s.n.], [s.l.], [s.a.] (preface 1551) (www.wul.waseda.ac.jp/kotenseki/html/ya09/ya09_00584_0019/index.html)

Rosenstein, N. Rosén von. *Underrättelser om barn-sjukdomar och deras botemedel* [*The Diseases of Children and their Remedies*]. Stockholm 1764; London 1776

Rosenstein, N. Rosén von. *Handleiding tot de kennis en geneezing van de ziekten der kinderen [...]* *vertaald, met aanteekeningen en byvoegselen vermeerderd door Eduard Sandifort.* van Cleef, 's-Gravenhage 1779

Schwabe, J.J. (ed.). *Allgemeine Historie der Reisen zu Wasser und Lande oder Sammlung aller Reisebeschreibungen, welche bis itzo in verschiedenen Sprachen von allen Völkern herausgegeben worden.* Vol. 11, Arkstee und Merkus, Leipzig 1753

Sesshū Hirano ō-ezu [Great Map of Hirano, Province Settsu]. Fujiya Chōbē, Ōsaka 1763 (facsimile print by Nakao Shōzendō, Ōsaka 1966)

Udagawa Genshin. *Shōni shobyō kanpō-chihō zensho [Standard Treatment Methods of Various Child Diseases].* [s.n.], [s.l.], 1845 (www.wul.waseda.ac.jp/kotenseki/html/bunko08/ bunko08_b0025)

Wú Juān. *Méihuāzhēn liáofǎ [Treatment Methods with the Plum Blossom Needle].* Běijīng, Zhōngguó zhōngyīyào chūbǎnshè 2002

Xuē Kǎi (author), Xuē Jǐ (ed.). *Bǎoyīng cuōyào [Compendium of Child Care].* [s.n.], [s.l.], [s.a.] (www.wul.waseda.ac.jp/kotenseki/html/ya09/ya09_00584_0009/index.html)

Yáng Jìzhōu. *Zhēnjiǔ dàchéng [Principles of Acupuncture and Moxibustion].* Japanese reprint, Edo Period (preface 1601)

Secondary literature

Chiba Tokuji, Ōtsu Tadao. *Mabiki to mizuko – kosodate no fōkuroā [Thinning Out and Water Children – The Folklore of Parenting].* Nōsan gyoson bunka-kyōkai, Tōkyō 1983

Deal, W.E. *Handbook to Life in Medieval and Early Modern Japan.* New York, Infobase Publishing 2006

Dore, R.P. *Education in Tokugawa Japan.* University of California Press, 1965

Herold, R. *Zur Sozialisation des Kindes im Japan der Tokugawa und Meiji era.* OAG, Tokyo 1992

Fujii Hideji. *Shōnishin ni kansuru kenkyū – shōnishin ketsuzō narabini ketsuatsu ni oyobosu jikkenteki kenkyū [Research on Paediatric Acupuncure].* Ōsaka Ikai-shi, 1927, 26, p. 3023

Fujii Hideji. *Shōnishin ni kansuru kenkyū – shōnishin ni kansuru chiken hoi.* Ōsaka Ikai-shi, 1929, 28, p. 3585

Fujii Hideji. *Shōnishin ni kansuru kenkyū [Research on Paediatric Acupuncture].* Imperial University of Ōsaka, 1930 (dissertation)

Fujii Hideji. *Shōnihari no riron to jissen (1) [Practice and Theory of Paediatric Acupuncture].* Tōhō igaku, 1940, 7, 10, pp. 28–29

Fujii Hideji. *Shōnihari no riron to jissen (2).* Tōhō igaku, 1940, 7, 11, pp. 32–33

Fujii Hideji. *Shōnihari ni tsuite no shirarezaru jikō [Facts about Paediatric Acupuncture Everyone Should Know].* Idō no Nihon, 1975, 34, 1, pp. 63–69

Fukase Yasuaki. *Shōnikagaku no shiteki hensen [Historic Development of Paediatric Science].* Shibunkaku Shuppan, Kyōto 2012

Hara Shimetarō. *Kyū ni kansuru igakuteki kenkyū [Medical Research on Moxibustion].* Kyūshū teikokudaigaku igakubu, Fukuoka 1929 (dissertation)

Kajitani Shinji. *Edo-jidai no ikujisho kara mita igaku no kindaika – Kuwata Ryūsai 'Aiiku sadan' no hankoku to kōsatsu [The Modernization of Medicine as Seen in Childcare Books from the Edo Period: A Transcription and Analysis of Kuwata Ryusai's Text 'Aiiku Sadan'].* The Teikyo Journal of Comparative Cultures, 2007, 20, pp. 65–118,

Kajitani Shinji. *Transformation of a Child Care Book Before and After Modernization – Commentary, Analysis and Transcription of Shōni Yōiku Kogane no Ishizue.* Teikyō Journal of Language Studies, 2010, 3, pp. 55–181

Kakinuma Masao. *Sugiyama kengyō denki* [*Biography of 'Schoolmaster' Sugiyama*]. Sugiyama kengyō itoku kenshōkai, Tōkyō 1980

Kornicki, P. *The Book in Japan – A Cultural History from the Beginnings to the Nineteenth Century.* Brill, Leiden 1998

LaFleur, W.R. *Liquid Life – Abortion and Buddhism.* Princeton University Press 1992

Nagano Hitoshi. *Nihon shōnishin-shi gaisetsu 1* [*Outline of the History of Paediatric Acupuncture*]. The Japanese Journal of Acupuncture and Manual Therapies, 2011, 70, 12, p. 106–109

Nagano Hitoshi. *Nihon shōnishin-shi gaisetsu 2.* The Japanese Journal of Acupuncture and Manual Therapies, 2012, 71, 1, pp. 264–273

Nagano Hitoshi. *Nihon shōnishin-shi gaisetsu 3.* The Japanese Journal of Acupuncture and Manual Therapies, 2012, 71, 2, pp. 83–90

Nagano Hitoshi, Takaoka Hiroshi. *Shōnishin no kigen ni tsuite – Shōnishinshi no tanjō to sono rekishiteki haikei* [*On the Origin of Paediatric Acupuncture*]. Journal of the Japan Society for Medical History, 2010, 56, 3, pp. 387–414

Netto, C. and Wagener, G. *Japanischer Humor.* F.A. Brockhaus, Leipzig 1901

Ōba Osamu. *Nicchū kōryū shiwa* [*On Japanese-Chinese Exchange*]. Nenshōsha, Ōsaka 2003

Ozaki Tomofumi, Yamaguchi Hajime, Yoneyama Sakae (ed.). *Jissen shōnihari-hō – kodomo no sukoyakana seichō e no apurōchi* [*Methods of Practical Paediatric Acupuncture*]. Ishiyaku Shuppan, Tōkyō 2012

Shuku Suteo. *Nihon shōnika ishi* [*History of Japanese Paediatrics*]. Nanzandō, Tōkyō 1964

Takashima Bun'ichi. *Hari no michi – naika-i no seishun* [*Way of the Needle – The Youth of an Internist*]. Shibunkaku Shuppan, Kyōto 2004

Tanioka Masanori. *Daishiryū-shōnishin – okugi to jissen* [*Paediatric Acupuncture in the Style of the Great Master – Core and Practice*]. Rikuzensha, Tōkyō 2005

Wernicke, T. *Shōnishin – Japanese Acupuncture for Children.* Elsevier, München 2009

Yokoyama Kōji. *Nihon kindai ikijisho mokuroku* [*List of Early Modern Child Care Books in Japan*]. Hōsei Journal of Sociology and Social Sciences, 2003, 550, 2, pp. 162–172

2

Introduction

2.1 Shōnishin and its development in Europe

Shōnishin in practice

The word *Shōnishin* first appears around 1537 in a Chinese text from the Ming era, being the name of a needle as fine as a single hair, used to lightly and gently prick the *azeketsu* ('ah-that's-it'!) points and *tsubos* (acupuncture points) in children.

As far as we can tell, Shōnishin did not become established as a non-puncturing treatment method until the beginning of the twentieth century (see section 1.8). As a result of one doctor's statement to the effect that methods of treatment that scarcely touched the skin could be more effective than the usual method of puncturing, the technique of gentle contact, which hitherto had not been taken seriously, gained increasing recognition as the 'right' one for treating children. He published an article about Shōnishin (the subject of his doctoral study in 1930) in an academic journal (Nagano 2012).

At this time families and schools of acupuncture had a monopoly of Shōnishin, since they had passed on knowledge of the healing art only in secret, from father to son, so that nothing could leak out into the public domain. So there was hardly any reciprocal exchange between individual schools and practices. There are said to have been instances where, in a form of 'industrial espionage', people would take their own or their relatives' children to Shōnishin practices with a good patient base, with the intention of covertly learning the art of treatment there (Wernicke 2009).

This politics of secrecy was not the case at the Daishi Hari School in Ōsaka. Masanori Tanioka, the Master of the Daishi Hari School in the third generation, ended the tradition of secrecy because, as he frequently says, the welfare of children is more important than reputation. Thanks to his untiring efforts, Shōnishin was able to spread not only within Japan but, from the end of the twentieth century, outside the country as well.

My first encounter with Shōnishin was when I met Masanori Tanioka in 2002, during a stay in Japan. Since then Shōnishin has been a main focus in my treatment of children – and there is a reason for this.

In the first weeks and months when I was starting to use Shōnishin, I couldn't really believe the results. Rather, I saw the improvement in the symptoms or condition of the children I was treating as a coincidence. 'The child would have got better anyway!' or 'Coincidentally, I was doing Shōnishin with him at the time!' So I thought, to begin with. It all seemed too easy, too simple. I was unwilling to believe that so much can be achieved with so little effort and technique! I wouldn't accept it. But so many coincidences – that just doesn't happen either!

At some point I accepted the fact that so much can indeed be achieved with so little. Since then, parents have regularly been coming to see me with their babies and children in the hope that I will give a Shōnishin treatment, either alongside a school medical treatment, or on its own. This meant that I had plenty of young patients and was able to gather a wealth of experience in this form of treatment that had previously been unknown to me.

…and in teaching

At the end of the 1980s my wife Karin and I set up *therapeuticum rhein-main* (Figure 2.1), a therapy centre near Frankfurt, with the main focus on children. In the years that followed, the centre developed as a point of contact for parents with children whose needs had attracted concern in all manner of ways: the newborn baby referred by the midwife after delivery; the small child with symptoms the local doctor noticed at check-up; the baby referred by the paediatrician at the hospital; children sent on the advice of their teachers.

In order to treat these children, doctors and therapists worked alongside one another at *therapeuticum rhein-main*. They all had joint expertise in academic medicine and Japanese methods of treatment, for example, Japanese acupuncture, Shiatsu or Sōtai.

The therapy centre is attached to a training centre, where the main focus for over 20 years has been the teaching of Shiatsu, with emphasis on Shiatsu for babies and children. After four years of intensive 'test-driving' Shōnishin in the therapy centre, in 2006 I offered Shōnishin training, based on the Daishi Hari School and the work of Tanioka-Sensei, at our training centre for the first time.

Since this first Shōnishin training got under way, interest has grown steadily among practitioners in different fields of therapy. In the first year we already had an inquiry from Austria about Shōnishin training. The following year saw the first training course in Vienna, where it still attracts a great deal of interest today. Two years later there were inquiries from Switzerland; since then, Shōnishin of the Daishi Hari School has regularly been taught there too. In 2013 a training course was held in England for the first time, and another will begin in Hungary in 2014. There have also been inquiries from Italy, Spain, the Netherlands, the Middle East, the USA and Australia.

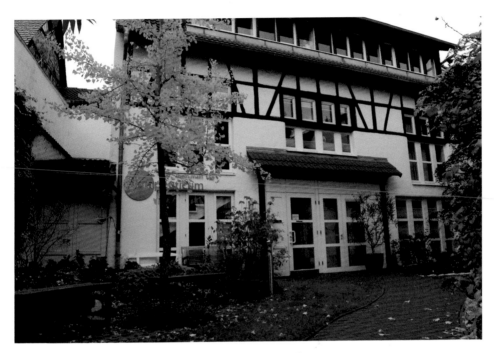

Figure 2.1: Therapeuticum rhein-main

The German publication of my book *Shōnishin: Japanese Acupuncture for Children* in 2009 – the first teaching manual on Shōnishin to appear outside Japan – certainly contributed to the spread of Shōnishin in countries where German is spoken. At the time I still had no idea what potential there was for Shōnishin as a method of treatment. Now doctors, too, are using Shōnishin at their surgeries – and latterly in clinics as well. As the reason for their increasing interest, doctors in general practice and in clinics say that Shōnishin is able to deal with problems in a holistic way and that the results speak for themselves.

Another probable reason for this development was that the many and various possible ways of using Shōnishin had not yet been exhaustively explored, so that even after publication of my first book on Shōnishin, I was still trying out the greatest variety of treatment techniques, quite a few of which I rejected – until in the end a few emerged from the process and passed the 'practice test'. In other words, anything that demonstrated a positive effect on the condition of children and adults, I kept as a viable approach to treatment.

Yet another reason for the spread of Shōnishin is the fact that this form of treatment can be applied by different specialist groups. Midwives, for example, are one such group. More than 50 per cent of all midwives in Germany already have some training in acupuncture. For midwives who do use acupuncture, Shōnishin opens up a new field of practice. For one thing, in addition to acupuncture with needles for women during pregnancy and childbirth, they can use Shōnishin if, for example, a woman has needle phobia. For another, they have an outstanding method of treatment which they can use to support the development of newborn babies. And last but not least, Shōnishin is 'portable' – wherever you go, you can take the toolkit with you, and treatment can be done anywhere.

However, it seems to me that the most important factor, and the reason for Shōnishin's increasing popularity with therapists and patients, is that it is one of only a very few treatment methods that deserve the 'child-friendly' label. For unlike most methods of paediatric treatment, this is not a treatment for adults that has been altered for use with children; on the contrary, it was developed in response to the needs of children, and exclusively for children. That is the essential difference between Shōnishin and other therapies for children, and it seems to be one of the secrets of Shōnishin.

2.2 The training

Training in Shōnishin varies a lot in the way it is done outside Japan. In Germany there are trainers who offer one-day courses. This, of course, entails the risk that therapists with minimal training could bring Shōnishin into public disrepute if they treat children outside their own household.

As a member of the Japanese Scientific Association of Shōnishin (*Nihon Shōni Hari Gakkai*), my aim in running courses is, first of all, to set a high quality standard, in the interest of both small and older children (Figure 2.2). It is based on current research on traditional Japanese medicine on the one hand and Western health sciences on the other, along with continuous development, by Karin and myself, of a model of energetic development (see Chapter 3). An important element of the training is the teaching of knowledge about child development from both Western and Eastern points of view (see section 3.1). Teaching on this subject matter requires lengthy advanced training and, in addition, regular continuing sessions (Figure 2.3).

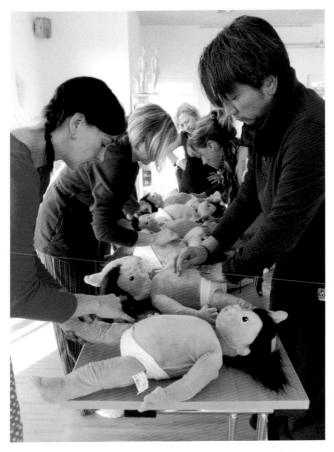

Figure 2.2: Course participants practising on dolls

Basic training in a meridian therapy (e.g. acupuncture, Tuina or Shiatsu) is a training requirement. In cooperation with Steinbeis University Berlin there is the possibility to gain certification in Shōnishin training.

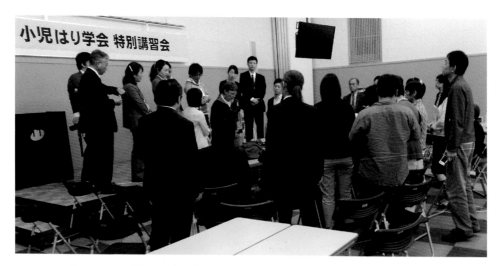

Figure 2.3: The author leading an advanced training course in Ōsaka

Teaching content

In the first part of the training the different treatment techniques, along with a basic general treatment, are taught and practised in great detail. Since, ultimately, children are going to be treated, the motor and sensory aspects of child development in the first 12 months of life are taught, as is energetic development. The most important thing is to understand how the meridians develop, and their influence on child development and development in later life.

In the second part of the training the main focus is on diagnosis and child development (motor, sensory, emotional and energetic development) up until the age of 6 and beyond, along with appropriate therapeutic procedures. Further, treatment strategies are worked out for selected diagnoses, such as bedwetting (enuresis), asymmetry in babies, bronchial asthma, etc. as well as treatment for adults. In order to obtain certification, individual case studies are required in addition to completion of training.

The great interest in Shōnishin as it is taught here rests on the theoretical foundation that underpins Shōnishin and baby and child Shiatsu. This foundation builds on the model of energetic development, which I shall describe in more detail in the next chapter.

3

Diagnostic Principles

3.1 The model of energetic development

From our practical work with children over the course of more than 25 years a model has emerged that can serve as the theoretical foundation for Shōnishin, and also for baby and child Shiatsu. We are talking here about a model of energetic development (Wernicke and Kalbantner-Wernicke 2009). It is the basis for understanding child development in its energetic aspect, and hence the basis for diagnostic and therapeutic processes that depend on the stages of development.

With this model we are attempting to bring the knowledge of modern neuroscience, developmental psychology and developmental physiology into harmony with the knowledge and experience of oriental medicine. The ability to assess children's behaviour correctly requires the gift of keen observation. Knowledge of sensorimotor development is also necessary.

The model of energetic development explains how, just like the stages of sensorimotor development, each stage of energetic development builds on a stage achieved previously. The meridians play a primary role in this. They represent a communications network connecting the child with her external world. Via this connection the meridians make possible, among other things, the integration both of reflexes and of stimuli affecting the child – and so they are also responsible for the development of a child's posture, movement, and patterns of personality and behaviour.

We can see by the many abnormalities that can arise in the case of disturbances how sensitive the interplay within the communications network is. Problems may become evident in, for example, difficulties with bonding, disturbances in perception, motor abnormalities or developmental delay, possibly to the point of a developmental disorder.

Knowing about the way motor, sensory and energetic functioning are interwoven opens up new perspectives on child development, from which specific treatment approaches result. Of particular interest here is the question of which meridian, or group of meridians, guides which stage of development.

Sensorimotor development from birth to school age

In order to recognise the interplay of motor, sensory and meridian development when treating children, one should be familiar with the most important stages of sensorimotor development from birth to age 6 and beyond. Building on this foundation, it will then be easier to understand energetic development.

I would like to begin with an initial overview of sensorimotor development in the first 12 months of life. More detailed descriptions of each of the developmental stages from birth to age 5 and 6–13 can be found in the relevant chapters.

If we split the first year of life into four quarters, then in regular development we can assume that by the end of each quarter at the latest, the following developmental stages are due:

- By the end of the first quarter, while lying on her back the baby is able to bring her hands and feet together above the mid-line of the body, with hands and feet touching (Figure 3.1). Lying on her front, the baby can raise her head when resting on her forearms (Figure 3.2).

- At the end of the second quarter, while lying on her back the baby is able to grab her feet in her hands (Figure 3.3). She can cross the mid-line of her body with her hands. She can roll from her back onto her front (Figure 3.4), and somewhat later from her tummy onto her back. When lying on her front she will use many different positions, between resting on her elbows and raising herself on her hands with her arms straight (Figures 3.5 and 3.6).

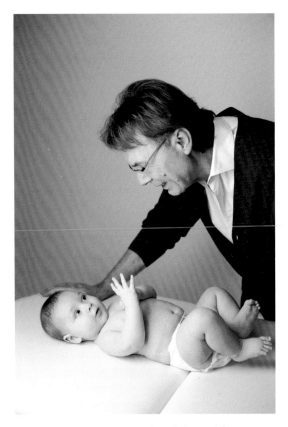

Figure 3.1: Hand-to-hand and foot-to-foot contact

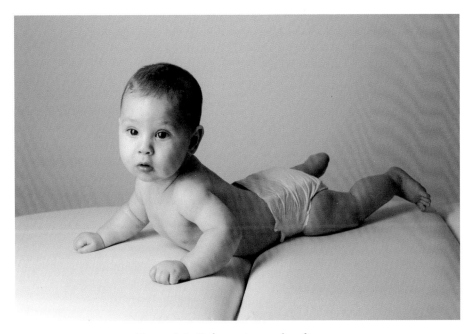

Figure 3.2: Baby resting on her forearms

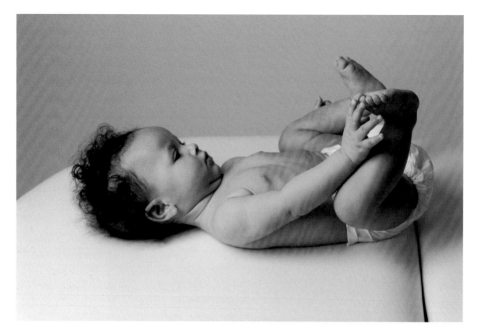

Figure 3.3: Hand-to-foot contact

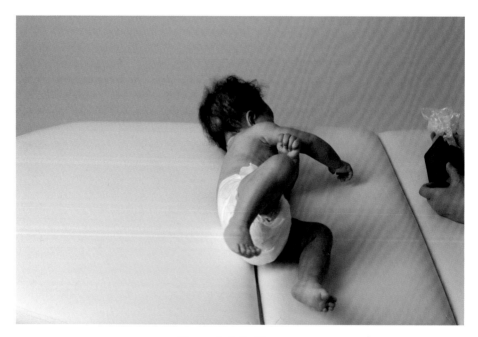

Figure 3.4: Rolling over

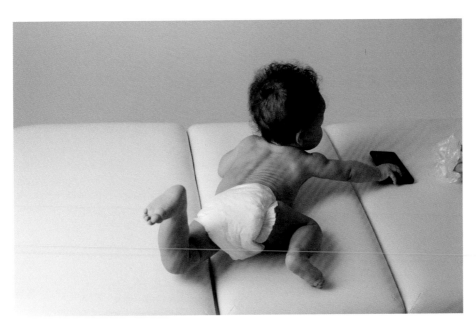

Figure 3.5: Leaning on one elbow

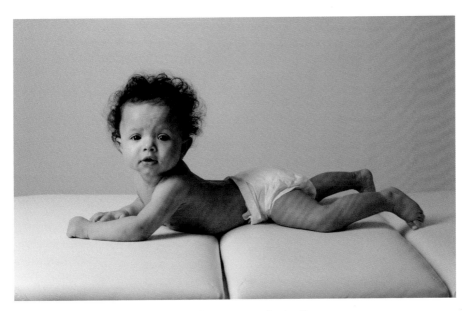

Figure 3.6: Resting on both elbows

- At the end of the third quarter she is beginning to pull herself along (like a seal), roll and crawl (Figure 3.7). She can sit down independently (Figure 3.8) and raise herself into a kneeling position. She is beginning to be afraid of strangers. She is developing great interest in details and small objects, pointing at tiny crumbs with her index finger and wanting to pick them up.

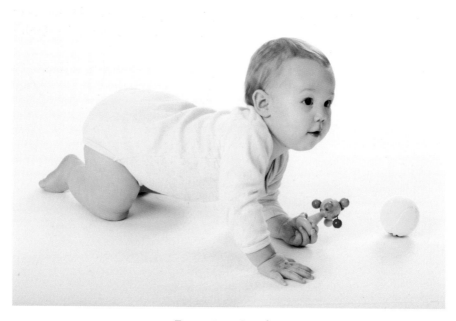

Figure 3.7: Crawling

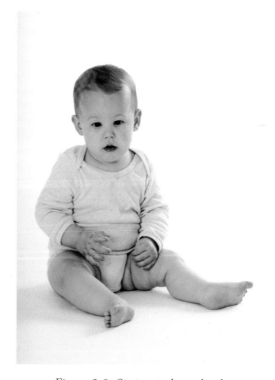

Figure 3.8: Sitting independently

- At the end of the fourth quarter the baby is at an intermediate stage between 'horizontal stability' and 'vertical instability'. She can pull herself up by holding onto large objects (Figures 3.9–3.11), and the first sideways steps alongside furniture are possible. The baby is beginning to crawl upstairs on her front.

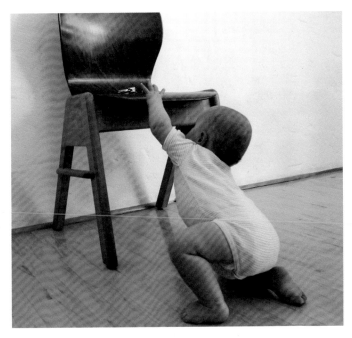

Figure 3.9: …discovering…

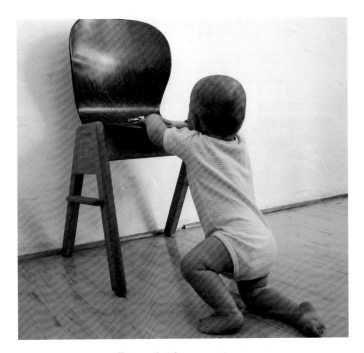

Figure 3.10: …steering…

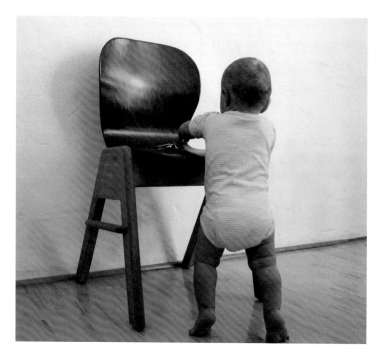

Figure 3.11: …triumphant…

In age-appropriate development the following stages should be expected in children between the ages of 18 months and 5 years.

- *18 months*: The child should be able to walk independently and to play for a certain amount of time. She can say 20 to 30 words, eat independently, and drink out of a glass.

- *2 years*: Now the child can move freely, and with good balance. She detaches herself increasingly from the caregiver and also plays with other children. Saying 'No!' takes on a central role. She can say up to 150 words.

- *3 years*: In walking and running, the movement sequence is confident and harmonious. The child can open and close a bottle. There is 'I' and 'you' – and a defiant phase.

- *4 years*: The child can stand on one leg for at least five seconds. Going freely up and downstairs is now possible. She knows the main colours, and every sentence begins with 'And then… And then…'

- *5 years*: The child can stand on one leg for at least 10 seconds, and also 'hop, skip and jump'. Now she can form grammatically correct sentences and talk about her experience in a logical, chronological sequence.

Meridian development: from three families to five phases

What is the relationship between sensorimotor development and meridian development? And how can we understand energetic development?

In the time immediately after birth, the human brain is not yet mature. But then, especially during the first four months, the brain develops rapidly. During this time the baby needs to have as many stimuli as possible, and as many experiences as possible, because these have an influence on the brain's structure and circuitry. The experiences that the baby has in these first months will have a decisive effect on later life.

In parallel with brain development, and the development in motor and sensory functioning that depends on it, we can assume that the meridians are also immature at the time of birth. In order for the meridians to emerge there is the same need of stimuli, to which the as yet unspecific meridians will (or will not) react in different ways. So the meridians mature by stages.

During the time after birth, this still undifferentiated system of meridians gradually starts to develop. From the existing undifferentiated 'meridian pool', three groups are formed. In each group, during the first year of life, four out of the twelve developing main meridians work closely together – so, overall, we can take three groups of four still undifferentiated meridians as our starting point.

In this early phase of life the meridians don't yet have separate existence, and so they have, as yet, no individual function. Rather, metaphorically speaking, each of the three groups speaks with a single voice. In the same way, each of the three groups has its special theme for life and development, and its particular relation to the relevant sensory systems – as remains the case throughout life. So as early as the first weeks and months of our life, the conditions are being set for the way we will later travel through life, and the lens through which we will view the world. In this way, in this early phase, the foundation is laid for continuing energetic development. We call these three groups or communities 'families', highlighting the functions of the three groups with their defining characteristics – in the same way as our family of origin is really our home, from which each family member receives the imprint that will last a lifetime.

Motor (as well as sensory) and energetic development are closely linked, for as long as the baby is unable to perform any goal-oriented movement there is no goal-oriented movement of energy in the immature meridians. This cannot be expected until the age of about 12 weeks. At around one year coordination and pattern of movement are sufficiently developed for the baby to be 'primed' to get up onto her feet. Likewise, the energy flow in the meridians will have developed to the point where it is following an ordered sequence within the meridians. Within each family the meridians are now linked up in a particular order, called a 'circuit'.

As the small child continues to develop, increasingly the separate meridians emerge within the three families. The fundamental transition from the four-legged to the two-legged state leads to a transition in the meridians communicating as circuits within their respective families – in parallel with the motor readjustment that is taking place within the musculoskeletal system. Now there is 'up and 'down' – the human being is standing between heaven and earth. At this point yin and yang come into play. The up-down connection of the related yin–yang meridians gives rise to the six axes or six *keiraku* that will be familiar from the literature on acupuncture. These start to develop at the onset of the walking stage and are fully developed by the age of 5 to 7 years. This means that during this phase of development the dominance of the meridians as 'circuits' diminishes and the *keiraku* increasingly come to the fore and determine development. A sign that the *keiraku* have matured might be, for example, that the child can stand for longer on one leg.

The older the child grows, the more differentiated and controlled she becomes in her emotional expression. At the age of 5 to 7 years a reorientation of a particularly psychosocial nature takes place, from the internal to the external (and vice versa). This also corresponds to the age of starting school in most countries in the world (i.e. by this point in time the child should be ready for school). Energetically this is made possible by the fact that the yin and corresponding yang meridians are all in synergy, resulting in the emergence of the five phases.

Only now – at the point of readiness for school – can we assume that the meridian system is fully developed. Accordingly, between birth and age 6 (and beyond) we can see three consecutive stages of development, which become evident in their different meridian constellations.

In summary, we can postulate that the musculoskeletal, sensory, emotional and meridian systems develop gradually from birth to age 6 (and beyond), with the next developmental step building on the previous one at each stage. What these four big developmental stages – families, circuits, *keiraku*, phases – look like individually, and what effect they have on the developing child, is explained below.

The three families

Let's take a closer look at the energetic developmental stages, beginning with the three families.

In the first year of life the meridians are at the beginning of their development, so they don't yet possess their individual meridian qualities. As separate meridians they are too weak, but collectively they give rise to the characteristics of the very young child – hence the concept of 'family'. So three families are formed, each with four meridians that gradually become specific. All of the four meridians belonging to each family have common qualities and main themes, so that all four meridians in a family can be seen as one big meridian.

Based on their location on the body, the families are called the front, back and lateral families. In the front family, the stomach, spleen, large intestine and lung meridians develop (from the second year of life: the front circuit); in the back family, the bladder, kidney, heart and small intestine meridians (the back circuit); and in the lateral family, the gallbladder, liver, pericardium and sanjiao meridians (the lateral circuit).

THE THEMES OF THE THREE FAMILIES

Each of the three families has its own special developmental and life themes. An overview of these will be given here. In addition, corresponding sensory systems are ascribed to the three families.

The front family

Developmental theme: Finding the centre

Life theme: Securing existence – Perceiving own boundaries – Ability to relate – Self-confidence

Immediately after birth the front family is responsible for meeting the basic needs of the newborn baby in order for her to continue developing physically and energetically, as now she is no longer receiving mother's blood. So the newborn has to rely on her own metabolism in order to survive, with a constant inflow of easily digestible nourishment, warmth, air and love, as well as undisturbed digestion. Here continuity is necessary, for the stomach and spleen meridians are not yet properly developed and cannot yet mediate between times of plenty and lack. Every interval in the flow of nourishment, warmth and love would weaken the child psychically as well as physically. In this case she could not develop resilience, nor her own foundation and stability – a long interval would not be compatible with life. In addition to the intake of nourishment, elimination of whatever is not required by the body is vital for existential support. Elimination includes stools, perspiration and the release of nitrogen.

The domain of the front family is predominantly the front (ventral) region of the body. Here lie the pathways of the related meridians that are gradually developing within this family. The front family receives the stimulation that is particular to it when the baby is lying on her tummy or being held in someone's arms (e.g. when breastfeeding).

A further theme of the front family is about finding the centre. That is to say, the head and hand-to-hand and foot-to-foot contact are on the mid-line. It is hand-to-hand contact that first arouses the baby's ability to reach towards something. Reaching in a targeted way always needs a starting point from which the movement proceeds and on which each movement is orientated – and that is one's own centre.

The sensory systems that belong to the front family are the tactile system (sense of touch), the sense of smell and the sense of taste. Disorders that may happen in this phase of energetic development mainly affect the digestive system, the skin and the immune system.

The back family

Developmental theme: Becoming upright – Getting moving – Language development – Auditory perception

Life theme: Setting limits at the back – Basic trust

Even a newborn baby is able to raise her head briefly when lying on her tummy. This puts her in a position to be able to turn it as well – so as to keep the airway free, for example. At around eight weeks the 'forearm rest' appears, which enables the baby to momentarily raise her head and turn it in a controlled way ('head control'). As development progresses, the infant gradually becomes more and more upright – initially resting on her elbows, then pushing herself up on her hands, then crawling and sitting, until finally the child is standing up, and ultimately walking. This period of development, from briefly lifting the head through forearm rest in the first weeks, up to the point of walking, is called 'straightening up'.

For this motor development the back (dorsal) region of the body is important. Here, already laid down and jointly operating, run the meridians of the back family; they will keep on developing within the framework of the child's development from 'four-legged' to 'two-legged'. At this stage the importance of the kidney meridian should not be underestimated (especially in the abdominal and thoracic sections of its path): it makes it possible to accomplish the 'straightening up' movement in an economical way, and inhibits over-extension during the process.

The proprioceptive system (depth perception) and auditory system (sense of hearing) are the two sensory systems belonging to the back family. Signs of disorders during this developmental stage concern the postural musculature, body tension and basic trust.

The lateral family

Developmental theme: Rotation – Flexibility – Coordination

Life theme: Ability to learn – Developing willpower

As the child develops the ability to turn, her willpower will also begin to develop. Now the child can investigate the space she inhabits more and more. The child can get close to things that were previously out of reach, and learn to recognise 'No!' which can occasionally lead to violent fits of rage and screaming.

Without the ability to turn, a child (and a grown-up too!) would not have the physiological ability to move. The ability to shorten or lengthen one side of the body is the precondition for the movement of rotation. Accordingly, the meridians that are gradually developing within the lateral family follow pathways along the outer (lateral) side of the body, and in the extremities along the inner (medial) side too.

The sensory systems of the lateral family are the vestibular system (sense of balance) and visual system (sense of sight) systems. Disorders of the lateral family can manifest as disturbances in balance and defects in rotation.

As soon as all basic abilities in each family are available to the baby, all three families can become involved in mutual exchange and interplay for the ensuing developmental stages.

Also, as the meridians become increasingly differentiated over the following years, the child – and the adult too – will refer back to the fundamental themes of the three families, again and again.

- So, on the energetic level, the front family provides the impulse to find one's centre, which concerns both the motor and the emotional realm.

- Most everyday movements are based on rotation. At the baby stage, rolling from the back onto the front, and later back onto the back, are the first expressions of rotation. The energetic impulse for this ability comes from the lateral family.

- The energetic precondition for the developmental step from frontal lying to the crawling position (or, as an adult, getting out of bed in the morning and also 'straightening up' inwardly) is met by the back family.

This account has presented the three families and their themes as separate entities, but it must not be forgotten that the three families are interlinked and interdependent, and influence one another in ways that may be either helpful or inhibiting. For basic abilities – for example, walking, sitting or jumping – the qualities of all three families are necessary. If a particular developmental step is due, then one of the three families becomes more active and comes to the fore.

Its temporary dominance does not mean, however, that the other two families are inactive.

The six *keiraku*

At the age of 12 to 18 months the child is becoming more and more upright; that is, leaving the horizontal, four-legged position behind and adopting a new posture. Now there is an 'up' and a 'down', and the growing child is moving between heaven (yang) and earth (yin).

This leads to a reorganisation of the meridians. The yin meridians of the front, back and lateral families of one arm form a unit with those of the leg on the same side of the body; as do the yang meridians of the arm and the leg on the same side. In this way, six up–down connections develop within the three families: three yin and three yang axes, called the six *keiraku* (meridians). Similar to the four meridians that jointly appear as one in the relevant family, the up–down connection should also be seen as a unit (yin arm–leg meridian or yang arm–leg meridian) – that is, as a *keiraku*. Here, too, we talk about front *keiraku*, back *keiraku* and lateral *keiraku*. This further evolution of the meridians brings the child to the next stage of energetic development.

In tandem with becoming upright, completely new possibilities of movement come into being, and therefore completely new possibilities for action. The child is now in a position (for example) to catch a ball while hopping on one leg. She can also rush round a corner and come to an abrupt stop if an obstacle gets in the way. In a similar way, the expansion of motor development leads to further development of the associated emotional and social themes.

If disorders occur in this phase of energetic development, the following motor abnormalities or abnormalities in perception and behaviour may result:

- Motor:
    - clumsiness
    - uneven movements
    - postural abnormality
    - avoidance of physical activity.
- Perception:
    - sensitive to touch
    - sensitive to noise
    - impaired balance
    - impaired body awareness.

- Behaviour:
  - fearful
  - clings to parents
  - constant fidgeting
  - tearful
  - aggressive.

The five phases

The 12 main meridians flow through organs, tissues, muscles and the nervous system, connect the body's internal biological system with the musculoskeletal system, and receive inputs from the environment, by means of which they influence organs, muscles, the nervous system and internal balance (e.g. the vegetative nervous system). At the same time the meridians support the flow of information between the motor and sensory centres while, conversely, movement and sensory stimuli reinforce the energy flow in the meridians.

The interaction of the information stream leads to the child being increasingly able to receive stimuli, make contact with her environment, react to her environment and communicate with it (Coenen 2011). In this way, alongside the up–down connection, an inner–outer linking of meridians forms within the three families – the five phases.

Through this inner–outer connection an increasing finely tuned power of emotional expression becomes possible, leading to an individual pattern of action and reaction. Whereas on the level of the *keiraku* the emotions are still very unfiltered and directly expressed (e.g. at the checkout in the supermarket a child throws herself on the floor, in front of all the customers, screaming in order to get something she wants), on reaching the level of the five phases the child has increasingly complex action and problem-solving strategies available to her.

Now the child should be in a position to express her emotions appropriately – that is, in a manner suitable for a given situation. She has gained the necessary social competencies and, with these, what we can call school readiness.

At this stage of energetic development in particular, motor abnormalities (postural problems), allergies, behavioural abnormalities and difficulties with attention, and also bedwetting, may appear. These abnormalities appear mainly because energetic development has stalled in the preceding *keiraku* phase, or in the 'three families' phase of development. For example, it is not unusual for a three-year-old child to fling herself on the floor because she can't have something she wants – everyone is familiar with it, at this age it happens time after time. But at school, throwing yourself on the floor and crying in front of your teacher and classmates because the teacher has forbidden you to play in lesson time can certainly no longer be considered adequate emotional expression.

Just like the three families and the six *keiraku,* the five phases have their own particular themes. If one of them suffers a disturbance, it can lead to symptoms that are typical for that phase. Here are the themes and the symptoms that may appear in case of disturbances, listed according to each phase.

WOOD

- Themes:
  - movement expression and movement planning
  - gross motor ability
  - coordination in movement.
- Possible symptoms in case of disturbance:
  - headaches
  - lack of flexibility in muscles
  - gross motor abnormalities
  - problems with balance
  - low frustration threshold.

FIRE

- Themes:
  - experiencing togetherness, sense of 'we/us'
  - pleasure in activity, capacity for enthusiasm
  - linguistic communication.
- Possible symptoms in case of disturbance:
  - insomnia
  - constant perspiration

- tiredness, restlessness

- red face

- speech and language problems.

Earth

- Themes:

  - attention

  - ability to concentrate

  - inner calm, finding one's centre.

- Possible symptoms in case of disturbance:

  - exhaustion

  - loose, flabby tissue

  - dry or sticky mouth

  - digestive problems

  - overweight, eating disorders.

Metal

- Themes:

  - perception of self and social competence

  - respect for personal boundaries (own and other people's)

  - capacity for acceptance, tolerance and recognition.

- Possible symptoms in case of disturbance:

  - problems in the respiratory system (asthma, bronchitis, dry cough, allergies)

  - sensitive skin, neurodermatitis, allergies

  - irregular bowel movements, constipation

  - sinusitis

- frequent colds

- over-familiar attitude and behaviour.

WATER

- Themes:

    - willing to take on situations

    - courageous in trying new things

    - ability to listen; relaxed.

- Possible symptoms in case of disturbance:

    - cystitis

    - postural problems, scoliosis

    - tense, tendency to overreact

    - lacking in stamina/endurance

    - problems with depth perception

    - restlessness.

Overview of energetic development

Energetic development happens in four phases, each of which merges seamlessly into the next.

- The first phase corresponds to the three families developmental phase. This begins before birth and becomes particularly evident during babyhood. Here each set of four undeveloped meridians in a family works as one. As in this phase their quality as separate meridians is still undeveloped; they speak – metaphorically – with one voice.

- The second phase is initiated by a directed flow of *ki* (Chinese *qi*) that is generated within the maturing meridians – triggered, in the first place, by the process of finding the centre. This leads to the separate meridians in each of the three families becoming increasingly linked with each other in a certain sequence – the three circuits. These appear at the toddler stage, and are capable of being used for therapeutic purposes.

- The third phase corresponds to the six *keiraku* developmental phase, which prevails from the point of becoming fully upright until age 5–7

- The fourth phase, the five phases developmental phase, begins at age 5–7 and emerges during childhood and youth.

Straightforward energetic development results in the child, young person or adult being always in a position to embrace each of the developmental levels described above, as the situation demands. To give an example:

I intend to climb Mount Everest (but as I don't ever intend to do this, you can tell that this is a hypothetical example). In order to get to grips with this purpose, I need inner confidence or trust that I am able to do it. This trust springs from the three families. The physical and motor capacity that I need in order to achieve the climb spring from the six *keiraku*. The vision and the implementation of the plan spring from the five phases.

The following graphs represent the development of the meridians – first, the collaboration of the meridians in accordance with the developmental phases (Figure 3.12), and second, the developmental phases from birth to adulthood (Figure 3.13).

Even though meridian development has been represented as a chronological sequence, this is not to say that each successive step of energetic development supersedes the one before. Each step builds on the last one, but each step of energetic development, once completed, remains in place (see Figure 3.13).

This means that as far as treatment at the meridian level is concerned, it should be in keeping with the appropriate phase of energetic development. Treatment done in keeping with the developmental phase will follow the flow of the meridian constellation that applies at that stage. For example, on the level of the three circuits this means that if the front circuit is the one concerned, then treatment will begin along the lung meridian, followed by large intestine, then stomach, and finally spleen (Lu → LI → St → Sp). The circuit is treated as a whole, and on both sides. If treatment is being done at the *keiraku* level, then the sequence for a *keiraku* condition in the domain of, for example, the back *keiraku*, will be kidney → heart (on both sides) and finally small intestine → bladder (again, on both sides).

3 Families

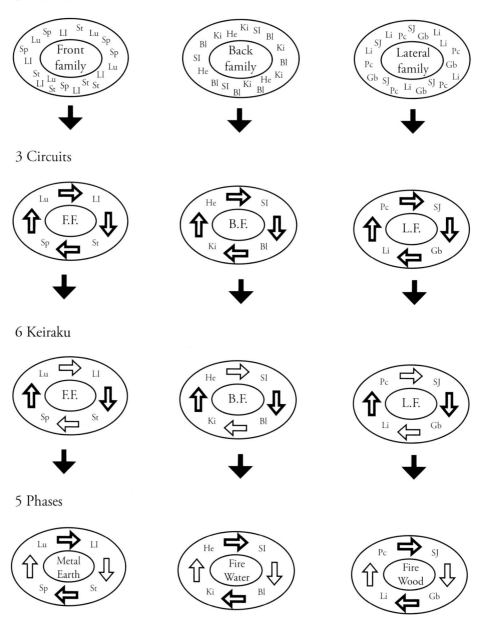

3 Circuits

6 Keiraku

5 Phases

Figure 3.12: Meridian development – the maturing meridians collaborate according to the developmental phases

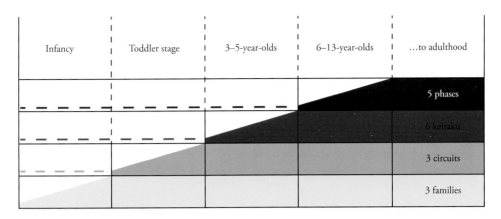

Figure 3.13: Meridian development – the developmental phases

Irrespective of biological age, then, the important question in treatment is, in which developmental phase did the condition in need of treatment arise? This need not (and for the most part will not) agree with biological age! The developmental phase that is treated is always the one that has not yet developed, or that has become stagnant. From this we can deduce the principles of treatment set out in the synopsis below.

Principles of treatment: an overview

- Three families developmental phase → basic treatment
- Three circuits developmental phase → meridian treatment of the appropriate circuit
- Six *keiraku* developmental phase → meridian treatment of the appropriate *keiraku*
- Five phases developmental phase → meridian treatment of the appropriate phase.

3.2 The surface of the body as the treatment zone

Besides the meridians there are, of course, scientific accounts of the way in which Shōnishin works. Here the organ we know as the skin, with its many qualities, has a special place within the framework of Shōnishin treatment. Shōnishin is done on the surface of the body, in a way that involves direct contact with the skin. The following sheds light on the significance of the skin as a sensory organ:

An orange. I can see the plump, round form, brilliant with colour, can stroke the cool, scarred surface. As I peel it I can feel the elastically connected, slightly brittle structure of the soft shell, and an invigorating perfume fills the room. Cool, slightly sticky juice drips from the fruit. I enjoy the sweet, slightly sour taste. Wellbeing spreads through my body. (Loebell 2012)

This is perception through all the senses. Images, sounds, smells, taste, warmth, pressure, speed, one's own posture, balance – all this penetrates into consciousness and is perceived. A requirement for this is sensory organs that make it possible to smell, see, hear, taste and feel. In order to orientate itself within its environment, the newborn baby uses not so much her hearing and as yet imperfect eyesight, but above all her sensitivity to smell, taste and touch. This last, sensitivity to touch, happens on the skin, the layer constituting both boundary and contact between the internal world and the external.

So the baby can feel contact and learn to 'grasp' the world through touch. By means of touch her also gains perception of herself. The infant's sensory experience is possible precisely because the baby's skin is so very sensitive to touch. Therefore, the skin as a sensory organ is hugely important for the development of the baby's mind, body and soul.

The skin as an organ of action – and reaction

At the embryonic stage of development the nervous system, the brain and the outermost layer of the skin (epidermis) are formed from the same cell material, the ectoderm. This common developmental origin explains the closely interwoven nature of the skin, nerves, brain and psyche.

And so the skin is an organ on and through which treatment methods like acupuncture, massage, Tuina, Gua Sha, cupping therapy and, of course, Shōnishin can take effect. In this way the skin represents a treatment zone that can be used for diagnosis as well as treatment. Neuro-anatomical and neurophysiological knowledge about the skin are not only useful for these methods of treatment, but also important if one is to be able to elicit a targeted effect by means of an acupuncture needle, hand, thumb or Shōnishin instrument. This is especially true of Shōnishin, which takes into account the different qualities of stimulation that reside in the specific characteristics of the skin.

As man's largest sensory organ the skin has the capacity to perceive sensations as different as touch, pressure, vibration, stretch, pain, warmth and cold. In order for this to be possible, a range of morphologically different nerve endings are needed.

For the sake of simplicity we can say that at the tactile level, over the surface of the body, sensory impressions coming from the outside are conducted further inwards. We are talking here about a *sensitive* system. The baby 'grasps' the world with its tactile sensory system, and in this way gets to know it. The *vegetative* system makes it possible for signals coming from the inside to bring about changes in delineated zones on the surface of the body (e.g. the 'Head zones').

Segmental sequencing

There is a close connection between the sensitive and the vegetative systems, such that the skin can both be used as an organ of action and at the same time seen as an organ of reaction: as an organ of reaction for diagnostic purposes, and as an organ of action for influencing the condition of internal organs or systems. The peripheral spinal nervous system and the vegetative nervous system make this complex interplay of action and reaction on the surface of the body possible.

It follows from this that disturbances in internal organs are projected onto the surface of the body. So areas of increased tension can be felt in tissues and muscles; using a sensitive tactile technique on the skin and the subcutaneous level, raised tension can be detected in the superficial layer of tissue; and likewise, increased muscle tension, by means of gentle pressure and palpation.

The figures below (adapted from Wancura-Kampik 2009) represent these projection zones on the anterior and posterior surface of the trunk.

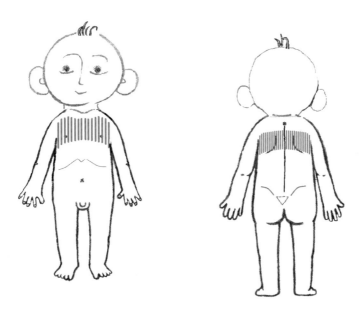

Figure 3.14: Lung projection zone

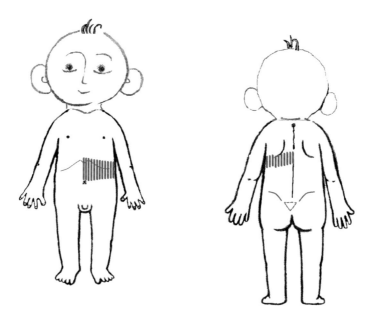

Figure 3.15: Stomach projection zone

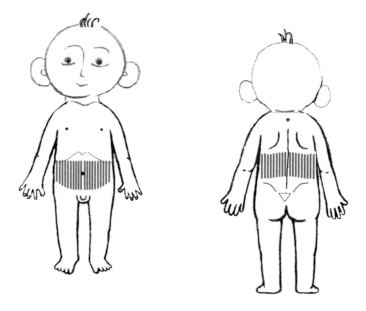

Figure 3.16: Small intestine projection zone

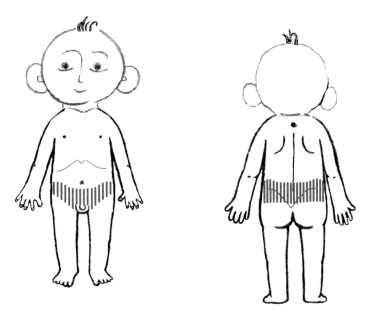

Figure 3.17: Large intestine projection zone

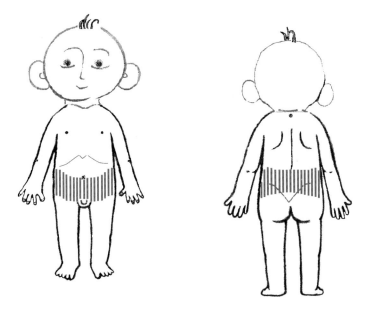

Figure 3.18: Kidney/bladder projection zone

It is interesting that these projection zones more or less match the reaction zones according to Masanori Tanioka (Figure 3.19). These zones can be detected by stroking gently. Tanioka puts it like this: 'One strokes as lightly as a feather, and finds states of tension at those points where the finger senses resistance or gets "stuck"' (Wernicke 2009).

Reactions in:

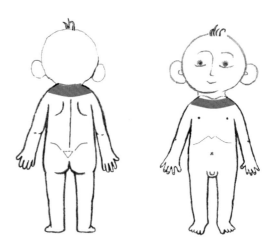

- *kanmushi* (crying, squeaky voice, biting, fearful at night, aggressiveness)

- common cold

- tonsillitis

- cough

- asthma.

Slight reactions in:

- loss of appetite

- unbalanced diet

- bringing up milk

- neurodermatitis.

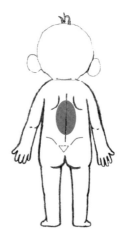

Reactions in:

- diarrhoea

- constipation.

Slight reactions in:

- bedwetting.

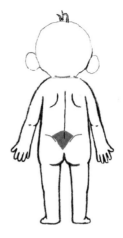

Reactions in:

- nervous twitching

- tics.

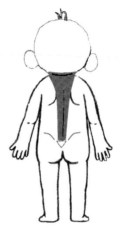

Figure 3.19: Reaction zones according to Masanori Tanioka

In the next chapter I shall attempt to show how Shōnishin works in terms of neurophysiological principles. If you are pushed for time you can skip this chapter for now without missing any important knowledge about Shōnishin, and read it later on.

Excursion into neurophysiology

Humans have 31 or 32 pairs of spinal nerves that branch off from the appropriate segments of the spinal cord. Each nerve pair facilitates interaction between its section of skin, muscle and bone and its internal organ – we are talking here about segmental sequencing.

The spinal nerves divide, mostly within the *foramen intervertebrale*, into five main branches: the *ramus ventralis, ramus dorsalis, ramus lateralis, ramus meningeus* and *rami communicantes*. The first-named three branches form the basis of a 'lengthwise division of the body's surface into three parts' (Wancura-Kampik 2009; Cranenburgh 2012) (Figure 3.20).

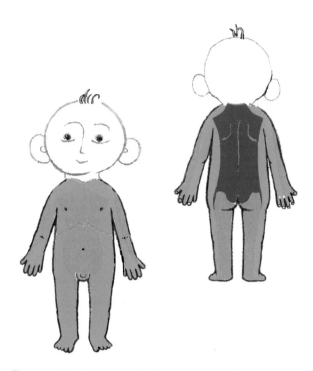

Figure 3.20: Areas supplied by the ventral (brown), dorsal (blue) and lateral (green) branches of spinal nerves

When we look at the areas supplied by the first-named three main branches, it is striking that the areas supplied by the *rami ventrales* more or less correspond to the domains of the front family, those of the *rami dorsales* to the domains of the back family, and those of the *rami laterales* to the domains of the lateral family. Here is the interface between neuro-anatomy and meridian thinking.

Shōnishin is, in the truest sense of the word, a 'superficial' method of treatment. That is to say, in contrast to classical acupuncture with needles, the skin is not penetrated during treatment, but work is done on the surface. Nevertheless, using different Shōnishin techniques it is possible to reach deeper layers in, and also below, the skin. There are techniques that are applied to the outermost level of the skin (epidermis and dermis), techniques that reach in deep (subcutis), and some techniques, the quality of which addresses certain nerve structures in the skin.

So a Shōnishin treatment that is done on a localised part of the body can have different results, depending on the depth of tissue addressed and the type of quality with which it is done – first, because certain qualities of stimulus are perceived only in certain layers of tissue (see Table 4.3), and second, because in different layers of tissue a stimulus will be conducted into different segments of the spinal cord, which in turn will lead to different responses to the stimulus.

MECHANO-RECEPTORS

The differing response to different stimulus qualities is made possible because the spinal nerves have different types of nerve endings at the superficial level of the body (Figure 3.21). The mechano-receptors (specialised cells receptive to specific stimuli) are one such group of nerve endings. Here there are specialised forms, facilitating perception of different stimulus qualities. Mechano-receptors, depending on what type they are, are located in different layers of the skin. The following are types of mechano-receptor:

- In the outermost layer of the skin, the epidermis (*stratum basale*), are the Merkel cells. They react to vertical pressure on the skin.

- Meissner's corpuscles, despite being in a deeper level of the skin (the dermis or *stratum papillare*), are nearer the skin surface than the Merkel cells. They register above all the speed of touch on the skin, and are therefore also called touch receptors. In areas of the skin that have hair the Meissner's corpuscles are replaced by hair-follicle receptors.

- Somewhat deeper in the dermis (*stratum reticulare*) are the Ruffini corpuscles. These are insensitive to pressure stimuli, but highly sensitive to horizontal pressure or stretching of the skin. So they react above all to pulling and stretching stimuli, which leads to reduced activity in the sympathetic nervous system.

- Pacinian corpuscles are located mainly in the deeper layer of the skin (subcutis), in the periosteum, joint capsules, tendons and fascia. They are vibration detectors, with a particularly low stimulation threshold. They serve the body as 'proprioceptive feedback' (Schleip 2004) (proprioception = depth perception).

- We should also mention free nerve endings, which can be found almost everywhere, but especially in the basal layers of the epidermis and in the dermis. About half of these have a high stimulation threshold, that is, these nerve endings react only to strong mechanical influence. The other half, the C-fibres, have a low stimulation threshold and respond to slight pressure stimuli, such as delicate stroking (Behrends 2010).

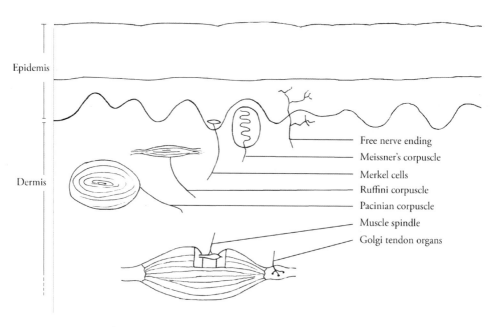

Epidemis

Dermis

Free nerve ending
Meissner's corpuscle
Merkel cells
Ruffini corpuscle
Pacinian corpuscle
Muscle spindle
Golgi tendon organs

Figure 3.21: Neuro-anatomical structure of the skin

PROPRIOCEPTORS

In addition to the mechano-receptor group, there is the group of proprioceptors. These are found not only in joint capsules and in muscle and tendon spindles, but also in subcutaneous tissue (the great layers of fascia lying close to the surface of the body), as well as on the surface of the skin. Their task is to keep the cerebellum informed about muscle tone (*tonus*) and the positions of the extremities and the joints.

VEGETATIVE REGULATION

The main task of the vegetative nervous system is to maintain the body's homeostasis under variable external conditions (homeostasis is the tendency of an organism to maintain a balanced and constant internal state). So this system plays an important role in the regulation of vital processes. It provides for regulation of rest and activity, and also mediates between sensations and the body.

Of particular interest are the effects of the sympathetic nervous system, which reacts to emotional and thought impulses. These sympathicotonic reactions can easily be observed, especially when the reaction manifests itself on the surface of the body – think of blushing in certain situations, changes in the moisture and temperature of the skin (under stress, for example), or localised goose-bumps.

Imbalance in the vegetative nervous system is caused mostly by overstimulation of the sympathetic nervous system. Especially in babies, who in the first weeks and months have not yet acquired a rhythm, the sympathetic nervous system is easily irritated. The vegetative imbalance this causes can be recognised by signs like crying for no apparent reason, being difficult to soothe, being jittery, having problems getting to sleep, not really getting into the deep sleep phase and therefore being wakeful, and having more wind – all signs of raised sympathetic nervous system activity.

Predominance of the parasympathetic nervous system may also be seen in the baby – although this is relatively rare. A parasympathicotonic reaction of this kind is apparent in reduced muscle tone, an abnormal amount of time spent sleeping, drowsiness while awake, and the baby in this state being extremely difficult to motivate.

Because the vegetative nervous system is noticeably more irritable in a baby than it is in older children or adults, it is also more strongly affected by the vegetative constitution of people who are close to the baby – which applies especially to the mother. Anyone who has dealt with babies in any way can observe how easily the mother's mood is transferred to her baby. This is also true of the Shōnishin acupuncturist! If he is feeling stressed, then he can pretty well forget about giving a good Shōnishin treatment – his stress will be transferred to the baby, who will react with restlessness or crying.

3.3 From the research on oxytocin

Shōnishin acupuncturists also observe that the child they are treating gets calmer and more relaxed with Shōnishin treatment.

We now know what causes this frequently observed physical and psychological effect. Swedish Professor Uvnäs-Moberg was able to show that among the free nerve endings referred to above, the C-nerve fibres, with their slow conductivity, respond to stimulation by delicate stroking (Uvnäs-Moberg 2005). The stimulus produced via these C-fibres is directed into the central nervous system, and leads to release of the hormone oxytocin in the hypothalamus. Here, in the hypothalamus, there is an overall control centre for the whole of the peripheral vegetative nervous system, stimulation of which leads to a generalised reaction throughout the body (Waldeyer 2003). In addition to the already known peripheral effect of oxytocin (contraction of the uterus in childbirth and orgasm, and contraction of the mammary ducts during lactation), a central effect, working directly on the amygdala, was proven. This part of the brain is responsible for emotional assessment of situations and social interactions.

With this, research on oxytocin established the far-reaching effect that oxytocin has on bonding and social relations. For example, after birth it stimulates maternal feeling for the newborn child (Deutzmann 2010). Oxytocin also plays a part in the fine-tuning of emotional states and appears to reduce anxiety and stress – independently of childbirth and breastfeeding. Because of its influence on social relations, and because it gives rise to feelings of happiness, oxytocin has been called the love and bonding hormone.

For the Shōnishin acupuncturist, this is one of the most important explanations for the success of the treatment; it also highlights one of the strengths of Shōnishin, namely the immediate reaction to treatment. In a child – the same, of course, being especially true for a baby – Shōnishin treatment has a balancing effect on the vegetative system, and is therefore a key factor in the maintenance or recovery of inner equilibrium.

Treating the child has a relaxing effect on the mother as well. Special nerve cells, the mirror neurons, are responsible for this. They are activated by the presence of other people and awaken the other person's feelings in the observer. The mother feels what her child is feeling, and in this way Shōnishin supports bonding between mother and child.

Part II

Practice

4

Treatment Principles

Preliminary note

The first contact with the child and the parents is used to gather information, using medical history and diagnostic procedures, but also to build trust on the part of all the participants. For this reason no treatment should be done on the first occasion, as the situation is alien for the child and this often makes it appear threatening. The child mostly doesn't know why she is here, or what is going to happen to her. And not least, the parents need to feel that they are placing their child 'in the right hands'. However, the most important thing is for the child herself to be able to trust the Shōnishin acupuncturist. Here success depends on mutual respect – and this is especially the case in dealing with the child, no matter their age. The first meeting lays the foundation for subsequent treatment.

4.1 Shōnishin instruments

We don't know exactly how many different Shōnishin instruments have been developed up to now. We can say with certainty that there are well over a hundred – the unknown total will be much higher. And the number increases year on year, with the latest developments mostly being made of plastic and intended for use by lay people in the domestic setting.

Figure 4.1 shows a small selection from the wide range of such instruments. They all serve the same purpose: to apply stimuli to the surface of the body by stroking, rubbing, tapping, scratching and applying pressure. Which instruments are used depends on which school of Shōnishin the therapist comes from. The origin of all the rubbing techniques that we know today was a mole's claw used as a 'rubbing needle' (Figure 4.2). This is still used today at the Tamada Acupuncture and Moxa Clinic in Ōsaka, which was established in 1927.

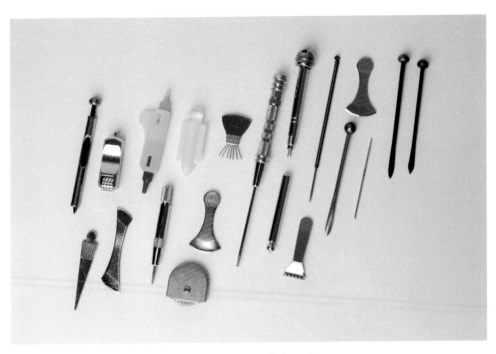

Figure 4.1: A small selection of Shōnishin instruments

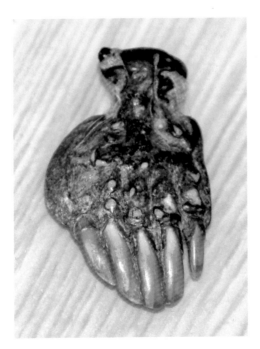

Figure 4.2: Mole's claw

4.2 Shōnishin treatment techniques

The form of Shōnishin used at the *therapeuticum rhein-main* is based on the Daishi Hari School of Masanori Tanioka (Tanioka 2005), the old master of Shōnishin. Here the Daishi instrument, which is rather like a nail (Figure 4.3), is used to perform stimulation all over the body.

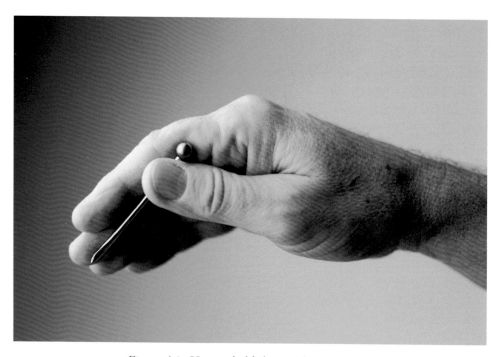

Figure 4.3: How to hold the Daishi instrument

Fundamental to the continuing development of Shōnishin techniques based on the Daishi Hari School is knowledge about the varied distribution of receptors in the surface region of the body. Here, account was taken of the different receptors, and with them the different modalities in the human body's response to surface stimuli. In practice, and taking the neurophysiological conditions into consideration, treatment techniques were put to the test, rejected or retained, in order to ensure adequate transmission of stimuli. As a result we use techniques that not only involve the meridians, acupuncture points or zones of the body, but also take stock of possible physiological reactions in the area under treatment (see section 3.2).

Not only treatment techniques but also the treatment instrument were adapted to the neurophysiological conditions. The deeper the nerve endings lie within the skin, the greater their receptive field (the zone that produces excitation of a sensory cell when stimulated). Nerve endings in the upper layers of the skin have a small receptive field. This means that the gentler (and nearer to the surface) the treatment on selected points, the more exact one has to be in placing the stimulus. This applies particularly to the vibration technique described below. For this purpose the Daishi instrument has been modified: its head, instead of flat, is spherical, ensuring that the vibration technique can be carried out with great precision. This has made it possible to achieve qualitative and quantitative variability of stimuli applied to different levels of the body's surface.

The classic stroking technique was augmented by four supplementary treatment techniques, all of which are done exclusively with the Daishi instrument. Of course, the different stimuli also can be done with other Shōnishin instruments, but using a single instrument like, for example, the Daishi instrument, has the advantage of not having to change instruments in order to place stimuli of different qualities, and so the treatment can 'flow' without significant interruptions.

The four treatment techniques that are used in addition to the stroking technique are:

- tapping in certain areas
- vibration on acupuncture points
- meridian stroking
- meridian tapping.

These techniques, using the Daishi instrument, are described below.

Stroking techniques

There are two kinds of stroking technique:

- first, the stroking technique as it is done within the framework of a basic treatment
- second, the meridian stroking technique.

BASIC STROKING TECHNIQUE

The basic stroking technique uses a light touch, and the frequency of stroking is dependent on age (Table 4.1). The resulting stimulus is very superficial, as the intensity of contact (which is also age dependent) is very slight. This stimulates the free nerve endings that are located all over the body, in areas both with and without hair. As around 50 per cent of these nerve endings react to light stroking thanks to their low stimulation threshold, the gentle stroking technique is the one most suitable for stimulating them. It is done within the framework of the basic treatment, which encompasses most of the body.

This stroking technique is also used to treat the projection zones described in the previous chapter, and also the areas around pressure-sensitive spinous processes (as described by Mackenzie 1921). The speed with which the individual strokes are done is registered by the Meissner's corpuscles mentioned above.

The following rates of stroking, which depend on the age of the child or adult, have been proven in practice.

Table 4.1: Rates of stroking, depending on age

Age	Strokes per minute
1–12 months	220–190
1–2 years	190–170
3–5 years	170–150
6–14 years	150–140
Adults	140–120

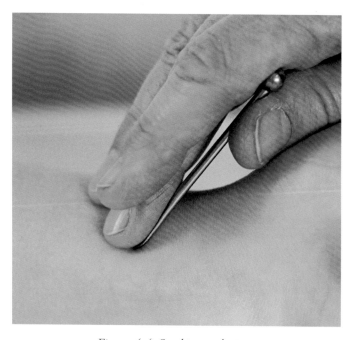

Figure 4.4: Stroking technique

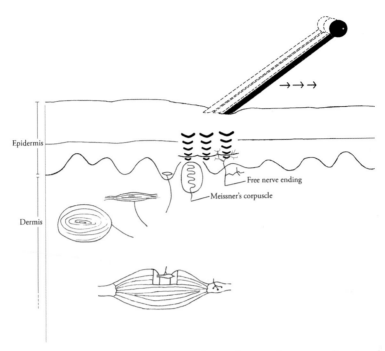

Epidermis

Free nerve ending

Meissner's corpuscle

Dermis

Figure 4.5: The connection between the stroking technique and optimal excitation of the free nerve endings and Meissner's corpuscles

Meridian stroking technique

To treat along the meridians, the meridian stroking technique is used. This differs from the distinctly gentler stroking technique described above, in that it is done with longer and more intensive strokes. This means that the main stimulus occurs not on the surface of the skin but in the region of the dermis. The longer and more intensive strokes produce horizontal stretching of the dermis, and hence stimulation of the Ruffini corpuscles that are located there.

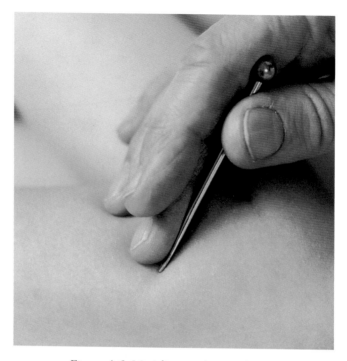

Figure 4.6: Meridian stroking technique

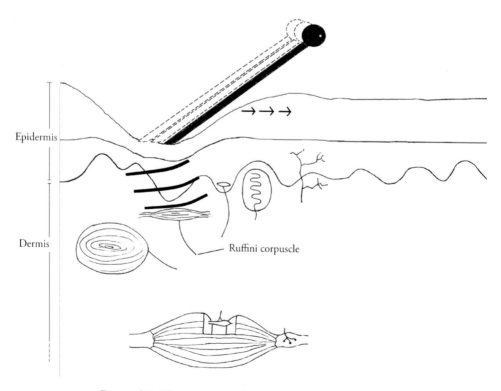

Figure 4.7: The connection between the meridian stroking technique and optimal excitation of the Ruffini corpuscles

Vibration technique

In addition to treatment by zones and along meridians, acupuncture points are also used within the paediatric framework. Most of these acupuncture points are in the distal, predominantly hairless region of the extremities, right by the bones and joints. The important main stimulation points of the related meridians are the source or yuan points (Table 4.2). In a baby, acupuncture points seem to emerge more like energetically denser areas which only appear in increasingly concentrated form as acupuncture points during the course of further energetic development. Nevertheless, these acupuncture areas can still be used for treatment purposes in babies.

Table 4.2: The yuan points of the 12 main meridians

Lung meridian	Lu 9	Large intestine meridian	LI 4
Stomach meridian	St 42	Spleen meridian	Sp 3
Heart meridian	He 7	Small intestine meridian	SI 4
Bladder meridian	Bl 64	Kidney meridian	Ki 3
Pericardium meridian	Pc 7	San Jiao meridian	SJ 4
Gallbladder meridian	Gb 40	Liver meridian	Li 3

For optimal stimulation of these points, once they have been located a gentle pressure is applied vertically to the surface of the skin with the head of the Daishi instrument. This creates initial tension, with the main pressure being on the subcutis or the bone. At this level of treatment the region of the acupuncture point is stimulated by means of the vibration technique, while the initial tension is maintained. Here in the subcutis, the periosteum or the joint capsule, are the Pacinian corpuscles, which react to the vibratory stimulus.

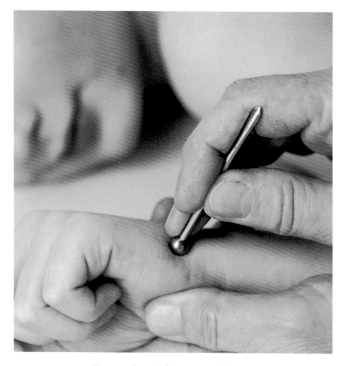

Figure 4.8: Vibration technique

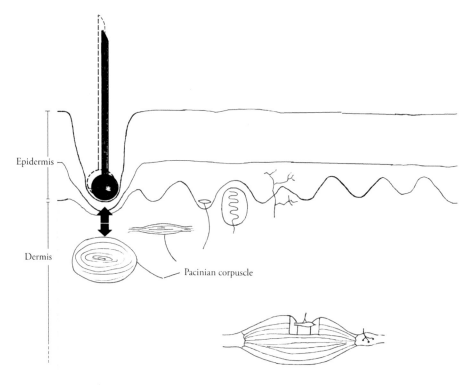

Epidermis

Dermis

Pacinian corpuscle

*Figure 4.9: The connection between the vibration technique
and optimal excitation of the Pacinian corpuscles*

Unlike treating adults, in whom stimulation of the yang meridian yuan points plays a lesser role because stimulation of yang is rarely necessary, in children we are dealing with a still incomplete meridian system. In them, stimulating the yuan points serves above all to support development of the meridians – including the yang meridians.

Tapping techniques

The tapping technique is used on certain areas of the body. Particular importance is placed on the tapping technique, not only for stimulating the particular regions of the body that are linked to the meridians, but also for encouraging the development of body awareness (proprioception). Four types are used:

- gentle, rapid tapping

- medium strong, slower tapping

- strong, slow tapping

- gentle tapping that produces swinging.

With gentle, rapid and thereby superficial tapping, it is mainly the mechanoreceptors that react, especially the Merkel cells.

Also, in certain regions of the body this type of tapping can lead to easing of tense lymph vessels, especially in the region of the lymph belt (Gleditsch 2002), as first described by Gleditsch in 1979. This region, which encircles the neck and upper thorax at the C4 segment, has an effect on the lymphatic and immune systems. Treating the lymph belt (Figures 4.10 and 4.11) improves blocked lymph flow in the head and neck, and has proved its worth in treating infections in the head region (mouth, jaw, ears, sinuses) and upper respiratory tract. Using the tapping technique in this area has also been shown to bring about improvement where there is a limited range of movement of the cervical spine.

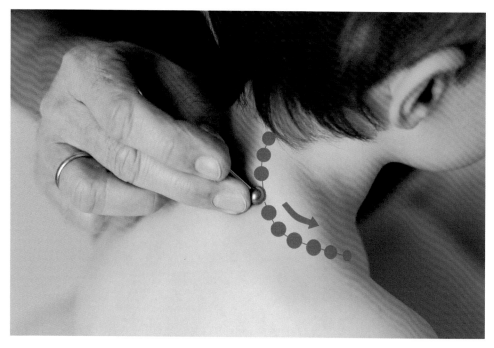

Figure 4.10a: Gentle, rapid tapping technique (neck/shoulder region)

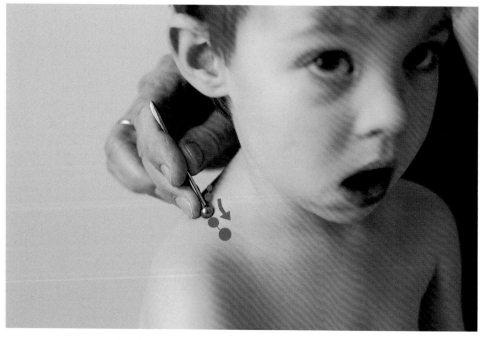

Figure 4.10b: Gentle, rapid tapping technique (shoulder region)

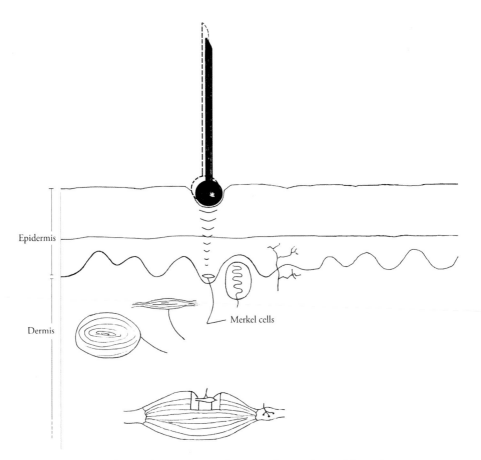

Figure 4.11: The connection between the gentle, rapid tapping technique and optimal excitation of the Merkel cells

Medium strong, slower tapping in the affected area stimulates the superficial and deep fascia of the neck, shoulder and upper thorax region. They react to this by relaxing. So we can see that the main uses of this tapping technique are for treating tension in the neck and shoulder area (Figure 4.12).

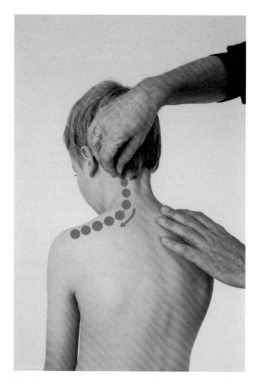

Figure 4.12a: Medium strong tapping in the region of the neck, shoulder…

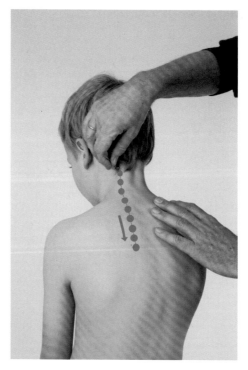

Figure 4.12b: …and upper thorax

Strong, slow and, thereby, deeper tapping (Figures 4.13 and 4.14) activates the muscle spindles and Golgi tendon organs and has more of an effect on the proprioceptive system.

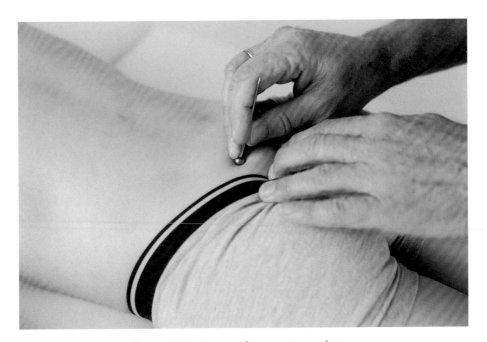

Figure 4.13: Strong, slow tapping technique

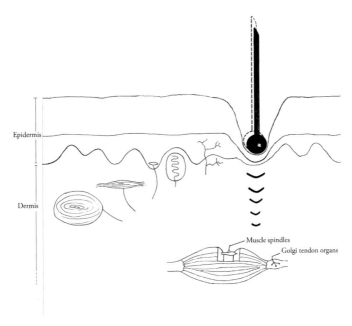

Figure 4.14: The connection between the strong, slow tapping technique and optimal excitation of the muscle spindles and Golgi tendon organs

Gentle tapping that produces swinging is a meridian tapping technique (Figure 4.15) that is used exclusively on the leg while treating the kidney meridian. It differs from the last two tapping techniques, most of all in its slow rate of tapping and slight strength of tapping. In contrast to the first-mentioned delicate, rapid tapping technique, the tapping strength of the meridian tapping technique is somewhat greater, but significantly slower.

In correct use of this treatment technique (which is done only in the frontal lying position), with appropriate strength and frequency of tapping, the leg that is being treated starts to vibrate and move with a rocking or swinging motion. The mode of tapping, together with the leg movement that it sets off, enables the patient to become aware of the kidney meridian deep into the pelvis and abdomen. The meridian tapping technique produces the impulse to become physically upright, so that infants lying on their front will be seen to raise their heads. In tandem with this there is an inner 'becoming upright'. On the neurophysiological level the meridian tapping technique stimulates the Merkel cells, muscle spindles and Golgi tendon organs located in this area.

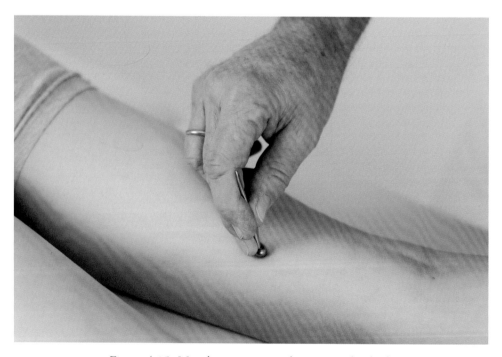

Figure 4.15: Meridian-tapping technique on the thigh, on the pathway of the kidney meridian

Table 4.3 provides a summary of the treatment techniques that have been identified so far.

Table 4.3: Treatment techniques and their neurophysiological correspondences

Treatment technique	Level of treatment	Receptor	Quality of touch (depending on age and constitution)	Frequency (depending on age and constitution)	Effect on...
Stroking technique	Epidermis/dermis	Free nerve endings (C-fibres) Meissner's corpuscles (hairless skin) Hair-follicle receptors (skin with hair)	Stroking (gentle touch) Pressure: 2–70g	120–220x/min.	Proprioception Vegetative system Release of oxytocin *Ki* dynamics
Meridian stroking technique	Dermis	Ruffini corpuscles	Stroking (intense) Pressure: 20–150g	60–80x/min.	Proprioception Inhibition of sympathetic nervous system Meridian system
Tapping technique (gentle)	Epidermis	Merkel cells	Tapping (gentle touch) Pressure: 10–50g	250–350x/min.	Tactile system Lymphatic system

continued

Table 4.3: Treatment techniques and their neurophysiological correspondences *continued*

Treatment technique	Level of treatment	Receptor	Quality of touch (depending on age and constitution)	Frequency (depending on age and constitution)	Effect on...
Tapping technique (medium)	Muscles, tendons, fascia		Tapping (medium strength) Pressure: 50–150g	200–250x/min.	Reduction of fascial and muscle tone
Tapping technique (strong)	Muscles, tendons, fascia	Muscle spindles Golgi tendon organs	Tapping (intensive) Pressure: > 150g	150–200x/min.	Reduction of muscle tone Proprioception
Meridian tapping technique	Muscles, tendons, fascia	Muscle spindles Golgi tendon organs Merkel cells	Tapping (gentle, rhythmic) Pressure: 20–60g	80–120x/min.	Proprioception Meridian system
Vibration technique	Subcutis, bone, joint capsules	Pacinian corpuscles	Vibration Pressure: 5–30g	400–1000x/min.	Tactile system Acupuncture point

Most of the techniques that have been presented here entail a stimulus so minimal that the lay person could hardly imagine such mini-stimuli having any therapeutic effect. Nevertheless, neurophysiology in the superficial region of the human body holds an explanation for how a therapeutic effect does take place.

4.3 Simultaneous diagnosis and treatment

More difficult to imagine is the rapidity with which the body reacts to surface stimulation. This is especially true of the stroking technique. After only a few strokes within the framework of a Shōnishin treatment, the experienced Shōnishin acupuncturist will note changes on the surface of the body that mirror the response of the vegetative system.

Watching a Shōnishin treatment, an acupuncturist who works in the 'classical' manner will observe an unusual process: palpation and therapeutic procedure being done at the same time. This simultaneous diagnosis and treatment looks like this:

The practitioner, while doing gentle strokes with the Daishi instrument on the surface of the skin, is simultaneously palpating with the fourth and little fingers of the treating hand and picking up on mostly instantaneous vegetative reactions – these are skin tension (turgor) (Wernicke 2009), reddening of the skin, skin temperature and moisture of the skin. For the practitioner these changes are important as signs that the treatment stimulus is being effective.

If we take a closer look at these alterations, we shall recognise the following characteristics and temporal sequence:

The first change to become evident is in skin tension. As soon as the state of tension in the skin changes (as a rule, by diminishing), stimulation here should not be continued. Continuation can rapidly lead to overstimulation of the area being treated at this point.

Certainly, a degree of experience is needed in order to perceive a surface reaction as subtle as a change in turgor – what is more, at the same time as giving the treatment; no easy task for a beginner! For those with less practice it is simpler, to begin with, to palpate the treatment area with the free hand before and after carrying out the stroking technique. This way, it's easier at first to concentrate on palpating.

As soon as the Shōnishin acupuncturist picks up on a change in skin tension – as a rule, raised tension returning to normal – he ceases treatment in the relevant area of the body.

A further change, which occurs sequentially after the change in skin tension, is reddening of the skin. When this appears it is a sign of incipient overstimulation – then in no circumstances should treatment be continued in this region. The same applies to all treatment techniques, but not to the intensive tapping technique, where reddening of the skin is desirable. A few Shōnishin schools in Japan do recommend the appearance of reddening skin within the framework of the stroking technique, but with no consensus on how this should be evaluated.

The last of the vegetative reactions to surface stimulation concern skin moisture and – in conjunction with it – skin temperature. If moisture increases (and at the same time the temperature falls), then overstimulation has already occurred and treatment should not be continued under any circumstances.

Of the three aforementioned reaction signs arising from the vegetative system, skin tension is the most sensitive and authentic indication of a body response within the framework of a Shōnishin treatment. The other two reactions – reddening, moisture and temperature – are uncertain signs, as they are very susceptible to the effects, for example, tight clothing or nappies in the area being treated. Only with touch that is sensitive to subtle skin changes, and instantaneous reaction, is it possible to give the optimal 'dose' of the treatment stimulus.

From the neurophysiological perspective, all the treatment techniques described here lead to the central nervous system (especially via the dorsal column) receiving information about the intensity and localisation of the vibration and touch sensations coming from the surface of the body, and the tone of muscles and tendons. Every single stimulus is conducted to the cerebrum, where it is processed, and leads, as a rule, to a motor or behavioural reaction.

Precisely in the first weeks and months of life, surface stimuli – like those produced by Shōnishin, for example – are important for the baby's development. Through the different qualities of touch in the various treatment techniques, the baby learns an increasingly accurate sense of her own body (which is still undifferentiated at the time of birth). So, through the different Shōnishin treatment techniques, she gains useful support for her sensorimotor development.

4.4 The permanent needle

In certain cases the additional use of permanent needles has proved its worth for treating children. These are available in different lengths, with a uniform diameter of 0.2mm.

The shortest needle is only 0.3mm long. As the skin (epidermis and dermis) is already about 1.2mm deep in a baby born at full term (compared to about 2.1mm in an adult), by virtue of its length this needle can only dip into the skin without fully penetrating it. If it is attached to a skin-friendly plaster, then secure application and no slipping out of place are guaranteed. The use of this needle is non-invasive and produces no feeling of discomfort or pain.

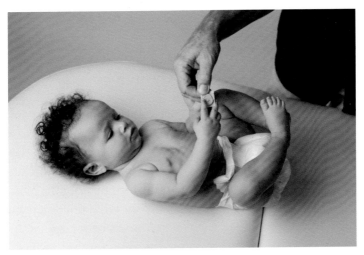

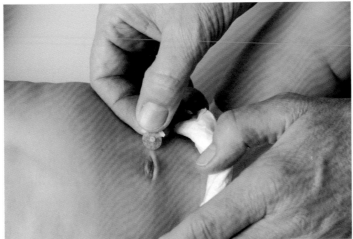

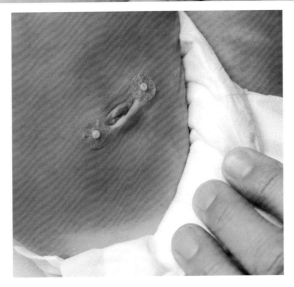

*Figure 4.16: Application of two permanent needles in
the St 25 area in a 6-month-old baby*

The permanent needle lends itself particularly well to the treatment of newborns, babies and young children (Figure 4.16) – as midwives also appreciate. The advantage of the short needle lies in the fact that even if it is placed in the nappy area (e.g. for digestive problems), the pressure of the nappy on the skin and the warm dampness under it will cause no irritation of any sort in this area. Even bathing and washing don't make the plaster come unstuck.

A further advantage is that, besides being painless to use, the parents can become involved in the therapy by gently massaging the needle in a circular motion – which can be done, for example, during a nappy change. After three days the parents can take the needle out by simply removing the plaster with the needle attached to it. If, contrary to expectation, a skin irritation should develop before the three days are up, then the plaster should be removed immediately.

Some symptoms, like hypertonic muscle tone, or the flexion contracture of the upper or lower extremities that may occur in cerebral palsy (the spastic form), require more intensive stimulation of particular acupuncture points, selected Ah-Shi-points or appropriate trigger points. Here, too, supplementary permanent needle therapy is an option in children aged over 3 or 4 years (Figure 4.17). It can be used, for example, to intensify the sedative effect by stimulating the appropriate acupuncture point, without reaching the point of overstimulation. In this case, application of the 0.6mm-long needle (which can also be used absolutely free of pain) has proved to be effective. After three to five days the needle should be removed – if continuation of permanent needle therapy is indicated, the needle can be replaced after an interval of three days.

The permanent needle is also a valuable aid in treating adults, as a complement to Shōnishin treatment – for example, in someone with low pain tolerance, or in adults with acute back pain who react very sensitively. Here the needles used are 0.9mm or 1.2mm in length. In general, 0.9mm or 1.2mm needles can be used in the neck and shoulder region and in the thoracic region without causing pain, thanks to the higher pain threshold here as compared to the low back. In the more sensitive lumbar region it is preferable to use permanent needles of 0.6mm or 0.9mm in length.

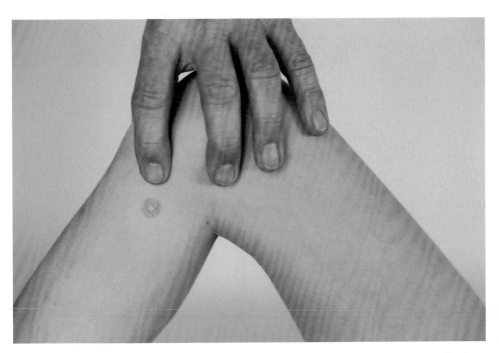

Figure 4.17: Permanent needle positioned at Sp 9 to relax the adductor muscles

4.5 General principles of treatment

Why should I give treatment as a Shōnishin acupuncturist? This question is meant not as a challenge, but rather to make the point that it is not always necessary to give treatment. The wish for treatment should therefore always be considered critically.

On the other hand, the Shōnishin acupuncturist should also be aware that a good deal of suffering can be avoided if treatment is given at the right time. Let's take KISS syndrome (Kinetic Imbalances due to Suboccipital Strain) as an example. What we have here is a crooked baby – crooked as a result of restricted mobility of the cervical spine (caused during childbirth). A functional defect like this is also called a 'blockage'. In many cases, with just a few Shōnishin treatments this lopsidedness will disappear. If left untreated it can lead to many symptoms, some of which may continue for the rest of the child's life.

If the Shōnishin acupuncturist does decide on treatment, then there are a few basic principles to consider in carrying out treatment and in the treatment plan. Let's first take a look at treatment in general – this means rhythm of treatment and clarity of stimulation.

Rhythm and clarity

Rhythmic movements have had a calming effect on babies since the beginning of time. The child in the womb is aware of her mother's rocking movement. In the sling, snuggled close to the mother's body and rocked to and fro as she walks, rocked gently in the cradle or lulled by the hum of the car engine – children love these rhythmical and rocking movements. In restless children too, rhythmical tapping on their back or bottom is an effective soothing method.

Rhythm is essential and plays an important role in treating children. This is especially true for babies. The younger they are, the more sensitive their response to rhythm and clarity of touch.

Rhythm means that treatment should as far as possible maintain a flow, and interruptions in the flow should be at a minimum. Each interruption in treatment can lead to irritation in the child, as experiencing a definite treatment sequence also means, for the child, becoming involved in the treatment. If the flow of treatment is interrupted, then to the child it can mean that the care being shown to her is being withdrawn. She becomes uneasy, and in some cases will give expression to the feeling. This applies in particular to the basic treatment that is described below.

Rhythm also means carrying out the relevant treatment technique with the child in question with an even level of intensity and frequency. This is true for the stroking technique, the vibration technique and the different kinds of tapping. In this way the child experiences stimulation that is clear, and the information that it conveys to the body is unambiguous. This clarity enables the body to react appropriately.

This last point contradicts Manaka's model of the treatment dose (Manaka 2004; Birch 2011). Regulating treatment dose by means of the stimulation dose neglects the fact that different intensities of treatment can produce different reactions. So one cannot assume that the speed with which the optimal treatment dose is obtained can be determined by varying degrees of intensity. Rather, different intensities of treatment will address different response systems within the body. The type of stimulation – and this includes the strength of treatment – determines which system in the body is addressed. It could be the endocrine system (e.g. oxytocin); it could be a reaction on the neurophysiological level (e.g. proprioceptors); it could be the energetic system (e.g. meridians).

Energetic age of development

In carrying out a Shōnishin treatment one has to consider that the actual age of the child and her energetic age of development are not always identical. Let's take the example of a child who is having problems with reading or writing. To begin with, it's important to find out where the cause of this weakness might be.

Is impaired hearing at the bottom of it, because the child has difficulty taking in and processing what she hears? Are there difficulties with seeing? Or with motor ability? Or does the problem lie somewhere else entirely, that is, on the psychological level?

The therapeutic process will be determined by the relevant *cause*, and by the *time* when the disorder that potentially caused the problem first appeared. If a temporal cause fits the picture – say, it was because the family had recently moved house and this involved the loss of a circle of friends – then the point at which the problem first appeared would be after age 6, which would mean that the therapeutic process for this child would be different than if the potential cause were a disorder of motor development.

Or let's take the example of excessive crying in babies. Here, in most cases the hidden cause is a blockage in the cervical spine – but only 'in most cases'. Tactile hypersensitivity is another potential cause. In that case the crying can be taken as expressing a tactile defence reaction. The treatment for excessive crying, then, should be according to the cause – in the first example it would be by releasing a blockage in the cervical spine, and in the second, by regulating the tactile system. For Shōnishin treatment that means two different modes of treatment!

The key factor that decides a Shōnishin treatment is therefore the age of energetic development. Accordingly, one has to determine the phase of energetic development during which a disorder or illness first occurred in a child. It is also necessary to know which family and which meridian (or meridians) are in charge of the related step in sensorimotor development, and what happens if a disorder arises at the corresponding level of the energetic-motor-sensory network. The child is then 'picked up' therapeutically at the developmental stage to which the presenting disorder can be traced.

So before treatment starts, the following two key questions have to be clarified:

1. At which developmental stage did the disorder or illness first appear?

    (3 families/3 circuits/6 keiraku/5 phases)

2. Which family, circuit, *keiraku* or phase is the potential cause of the disorder or illness?

    (front, back or lateral family/circuit/keiraku or appropriate phase)

The answers to these two questions produce the treatment strategy. That is, the child will be treated:

1. at the level of the family, circuit, *keiraku* or phase, and

2. within the domain of the front, back or lateral family/circuit/*keiraku* or appropriate phase.

This knowledge forms the foundation for treating children of any age with Shōnishin.

The following graphs show examples of disorders occurring at different stages of energetic development. Here it is easy to see that the biological age and the underlying energetic disorder don't necessarily arise from the same developmental stage, in either a child or an adult.

EXAMPLE 1

A 4-year-old displays clear patterns of motor, emotional or social behaviour that are typically seen in toddlers. Therefore treatment must be done at the level at which development stalled – in this case, the toddler level. Accordingly, the front, back or lateral circuit is treated.

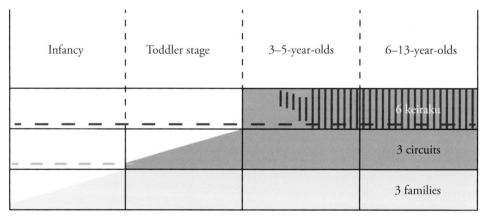

Figure 4.18: A 4-year-old child shows symptoms or disorders originating at the toddler stage

EXAMPLE 2

A child of 9 years displays clear patterns of motor, emotional or social behaviour that are typically seen in toddlers. Here, too, treatment must be done at the toddler level. Accordingly, the front, back or lateral circuit is treated, so that the next step in development, the undisturbed emergence of the *keiraku*, can be completed.

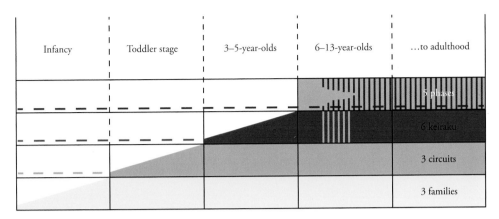

Figure 4.19: A child aged 9 years shows symptoms or disorders originating at the toddler stage

EXAMPLE 3

If a child of 12 years displays motor, emotional or social patterns that are to be expected in younger children but not in children aged 12 years, then the child is treated at the appropriate energetic level – the one at which development stalled. In this case the *keiraku* level would need support for the next step in development, the emergence of the five phases, to take place.

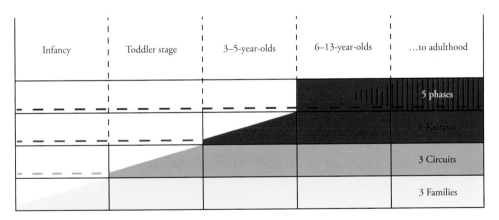

Figure 4.20: A child aged 12 years shows symptoms or disorders originating at the 3–5-year-old stage

4.6 Indications and contraindications

Indications for Shōnishin treatment

Depending on the Shōnishin acupuncturist's professional background, their patient group and the indications associated with it will vary. The professional groups set out below are intended as examples. In all cases, training in acupuncture or Shiatsu, or traditional Japanese or Chinese medicine, is taken for granted as a precondition for practising Shōnishin:

- *Paediatricians* mainly treat infants with problems of the digestive tract or respiratory organs, and young and older children with developmental disorders.

- *General practitioners* treat children with behavioural abnormalities at nursery school and those with poor concentration and ADD/ADHD at school, as well as children with neurodermatitis, bronchial asthma and bedwetting problems. If they use Shōnishin with adults, in many cases these are adults with needle phobia or sensitive reactions, or very old people (e.g. on anticoagulants).

- *Orthopaedists* use Shōnishin mainly with children with postural or musculoskeletal problems.

- *Midwives* naturally deal with newborns. Here Shōnishin's greatest value is in supporting babies who cry excessively. Shōnishin has also proved its worth for drinking problems or tummy ache (three-month colic), to name only the most important indications, and many midwives could not imagine practising without it. Women in pregnancy and childbirth are another target group for midwives. For them Shōnishin can be used successfully in preparation for childbirth and, following delivery, for support with postnatal weakness or blocked milk ducts.

- *Shiatsu practitioners* like to use Shōnishin as a complement to baby or child Shiatsu, for developmental support.

- *Physiotherapists* have found an improved success rate in the treatment of children with cerebral palsy because supplementary Shōnishin treatment helps to reduce the often increased muscle tone in these children.

- *Occupational therapists* and *speech therapists* use Shōnishin as an aid to development of better body awareness, making for more effective delivery of therapy.

- *Osteopaths* and *chiropractors* have discovered Shōnishin as an integral component of treatment of asymmetrical babies (KISS babies), because complementary treatment with Shōnishin significantly reduces the incidence of relapse in the babies treated (renewed occurrence of a blockage after successful treatment) (Kalbantner-Wernicke and Wernicke 2010).

The following information refers to my work at *therapeuticum rhein-main*, where the most frequent reasons for seeking Shōnishin treatment are the following:

- *Babies*: excessive crying, KISS syndrome, three-month colic, feeding problems, sleep disturbance, support for mother–child bonding.

- *Toddlers*: sleep disturbance, eating problems, digestive ailments (colic, diarrhoea, constipation), neurodermatitis, bronchitis, epilepsy, developmental delay.

- *3–5-year-olds*: susceptibility to infection, motor abnormality, obstructive bronchitis, inflammation of the middle ear, neurodermatitis, cerebral palsy, epilepsy, perceptual/behavioural abnormalities, developmental delay.

- *6–13-year-olds*: postural problems, headache, ADD, ADHD, susceptibility to infection, perceptual/behavioural abnormalities, bronchial asthma, allergies, bedwetting, cerebral palsy, epilepsy.

- *Adults*: needle phobia, hypersensitive reaction to acupuncture treatment; *in combination with acupuncture/manual treatment methods*: prenatal care, blocked milk ducts, scarring.

- *Older people*: dementia, multimorbidity, isolation.

Contraindications

Alongside contraindications that hardly need mentioning, because they fall under the remit of medical specialists (bone fractures, fresh wounds, loss of consciousness, seizures, difficulty breathing or sudden pallor), the following conditions or illnesses should be included in the list of contraindications.

FEVER

When the body temperature rises above 38.5°C, we are talking of fever. Although high temperature is not an illness but a reaction to illness, children should not be treated with Shōnishin for the purpose of speeding recovery. Even a treatment method as gentle as Shōnishin instantly leads to overstimulation in the fevered state, because of heightened sensitivity to touch.

INFECTIOUS ILLNESSES

Infectious illnesses are caused as a rule by viruses, bacteria or fungi. Many of these pathogens are harmless, while others make the child feel very ill. In the latter case the sick child feels weak, is more or less sensitive to external stimuli and is often running a temperature. As the skin is usually hypersensitive in a feverish child, she does not like to be touched. She wants to be left in peace – which makes sense, as rest is the most effective therapy, especially for avoiding complications.

As for infectious illnesses, one should be aware that some of them are highly infectious. Children with measles or chickenpox should therefore not go outside their home environment – they don't feel like it anyway. They feel – and this applies especially to measles – really poorly.

For these reasons, doing a Shōnishin treatment or even acupuncture with needles is out of the question, even if relevant specialist literature recommends doing acupuncture on children with infectious illnesses. For example, Flaws (2007) recommends 'let[ting] a few drops of blood at several points' in cases of measles, and Scott and Barlow (2008) – also with reference to measles – writes 'It may be that they [the children] don't want acupuncture, but this resistance is easier to break down.'

However, Shōnishin treatment should be weighed critically, and not only if the child has an infectious illness – an acute illness such as influenza, herpes or shingles in the parents is also a contraindication. And naturally the same applies if the Shōnishin acupuncturist has a cold or an infectious illness.

IMMUNISATION

While this does not mean an illness, an immunisation given less than four days previously is also a contraindication. Whether or not there is a temperature, immunisation means that the young body is having to get to grips with a weakened pathogen. It is busy enough with that. If, during this phase, a Shōnishin treatment were to be done as well, then the body would be affected by receiving too much input in too short a time. This can easily overload the body and lead, in some cases, to undesirable side effects.

HEAD LICE

Head lice aren't painful – but they get on your nerves! Contrary to widespread belief, they have nothing to do with poor standards of personal cleanliness – they very much like freshly washed hair (or even especially).

Head lice brought into the practice by a child leads to complicated cleaning of upholstered surfaces on which the child lay and, where applicable, of soft toys the child played with. Upholstery, towels and suchlike are machine-washed at a temperature of at least 60°C, and then preferably dried in a tumble-drier. Soft toys that would not survive heat treatment are put into a plastic sack with a secure closure and put into the freezer for 24 hours.

STUBBORN REFUSAL ON THE PART OF THE CHILD

A child who fights tooth and nail against Shōnishin treatment should not be treated. Even if the treatment were for the good of the child, the Shōnishin acupuncturist should always respect the child's resistance. It generally happens (if at all) before the first treatment. The child may have had painful experiences, or have been 'shown' to several therapists already – there are plenty of reasons for resisting.

A child behaving like this is usually around the age of 2 or 3. As Shōnishin is not being used as a life-saving therapy in cases like this, it is fine to wait and make another appointment for a few weeks' or months' time (should the problem still require attention by then).

It's different with babies. Here it's a matter of being prompt to spot expressions of feeling, interpreting them correctly and responding appropriately – these are essential requirements if the Shōnishin acupuncturist is to be able to carry out successful treatment. From modern research on infants we know that babies express their internal state from the first moment of their lives. If they are sad or cross, they show it; they show pleasure if they like something, and they also show rejection and refusal. It is especially important to recognise defensive reactions in particular, and all the more because a baby is able to display a multitude of defensive reactions. These may be expressed by the baby's body bracing itself, or by avoidance postures, such as avoiding eye contact with the practitioner, or evasive body movements. The defensive reactions may become heightened, from the baby pushing the practitioner's hand away, to a general state of hyperarousal expressed by first whimpering, then crying, and finally screaming.

Spotting these signs, and a prompt response on the practitioner's part, will save the situation in many cases, so that after a short interval the treatment can be resumed. Ignoring these stress signals inevitably ends with abandoning treatment!

4.7 Signs of overstimulation

Children are more easily stimulated by treatment than adults are, and by the same token they are also more easily overstimulated. This is not only because their *ki* dynamics have a strong yang character (see section 5.2), but also because their reactions have not yet become inflexible due to heavy metals, traumatic experiences, electro smog, etc. Toddlers and babies react with particular sensitivity, so with them the point of overstimulation is quickly reached.

To avoid jeopardising successful treatment it is most important to recognise overstimulation in time – this applies especially to babies and toddlers. The most frequent causes of overstimulation are:

- treating for too long

- using too many different stimuli during one session

- the effect on the child of too many stimuli in her immediate surroundings.

Treating for too long

The length of treatment for babies and toddlers should not exceed 5 to 10 minutes – unless the treatment is interspersed with breaks or a rest. Once they have been treated for a maximum of 15 minutes, babies and toddlers have reached the limit of their receptivity. More treatment will lead to defensive reactions.

Using too many different stimuli during one session

Often the practitioner is tempted to 'pull out all the stops' in an attempt to achieve the best possible treatment. But for the child this means exposure to a multitude of different stimuli. Then treatment input loses clarity, depriving the body of the chance to react clearly. The clearer the information the child receives from the treatment input, the better she is able to assimilate and process this input.

The effect on the child of too many stimuli in her immediate surroundings

A restful environment is very important when treating a child. Anxiety has a negative effect on the child who has come for treatment, as it easily rubs off on the child. Causes of anxiety might be:

- the mother or father coming to the appointment in a rush

- mother or father giving off anxiety themselves

- mother or father always offering action to the child

- a whimpering sibling is present

- the practitioner is anxious because of time pressure, uncertain about the parents, distracted by personal matters, etc.

While children will clearly indicate or say when they have had enough, babies express their need for a break or show that they have had enough through signs or their behaviour. If overstimulated, babies will, as a rule, react according to the following pattern.

If she needs a break or time to process the large number of impressions, the baby first breaks eye contact with the practitioner. If treatment continues regardless, the baby will become restless and withdraw her arms and legs. Soon after that she will start to make herself more and more stiff, her breathing rate increases, she starts to perspire and begins whimpering, which very is very soon amplified to crying and finally to screaming.

For the most part, the different phases that the baby goes through will occur very swiftly, one after the other – sometimes so fast that they appear to be happening almost all at the same time. How and when these signs appear, however, is impossible to predict; the sequence is individual and may vary a lot, depending on the situation. Many babies avert their gaze and immediately begin to scream at the tops of their voices; others send out numerous warning signals before making their message clear. With a bit of experience you get to see the signs in good time, before the baby reaches the point of having to express them.

The practitioner will hear about the consequences of overstimulation at the next appointment – as, foreseeably, the mother or father will report that, following treatment, their baby was feeble and tired, or slept for a remarkably long time. In some circumstances, from the age of 2 to 3 years and upwards, children may react with hyperactivity. If the child was treated for pain, the parents occasionally report that the pain was temporarily worse. A further sign of overstimulation could be a temporary rise in temperature.

4.8 Difficult situations

Crying

Children who cry or put up resistance cannot be treated (see section 4.6). The exception is babies who cry excessively – you cannot expect them *not* to cry at the moment they are about to be treated. No matter what the reason for crying, they are in an exceptional, dysregulated vegetative state that makes them extremely irritable, and therefore hypersensitive to any external stimulus.

Treatment for a baby who cries excessively is, therefore, quick and possibly shorter than usual, and in some cases may be done with the baby lying only on her back, or only on her front.

Fear of strangers

In order to treat a baby who is afraid of strangers, one important principle in Shōnishin is disregarded. This principle states that when treating a child – and this applies especially to babies – constant eye contact should be maintained. With a baby or small child who is afraid of strangers, this inevitably makes her cry so that this principle (exceptionally!) does not apply.

Instead, act as if you are not interested in the child and talk only with the mother or father about anything at all, except about the child. This way, the treatment is done 'incidentally'. While treating the child, the Shōnishin acupuncturist observes her out of the corner of his eye, so as to be able to respond sufficiently to any defensive behaviour on the child's part.

Defiance

The defiance phase is a challenge, not just for parents but also for any therapist involved. Paediatricians could tell you about it until the cows come home! If a child in the defiance phase doesn't want to be treated, she doesn't want to. No way! Cajoling will get you nowhere; bribery rarely bears fruit. (For more on this see section 4.6.)

Fearfulness

Again and again in the context of the first Shōnishin treatment, you will be faced with a child who is scared. This fear frequently stems from the fact that the child has already been shown to all kinds of adults on account of certain abnormalities. What experiences has she had during the process?

In practice it looks something like this: At nursery the teacher takes Ben's mother on one side and tells her, with Ben standing next to his mother, 'I think there is something the matter with Ben – he always looks so clumsy when he's running – aren't you, Ben? Today you tripped over your own feet again!' And then in the evening, when father comes home from work: 'Let Daddy see you running – his kindergarten teacher spoke to me today about the funny way he runs! We'll have to do something about it.'

The following evening when his parents have invited friends to tea, naturally and inevitably everyone starts talking about their children. 'Ben? Where are you? Come here and show Paula and Sven how you run. They've even noticed it at nursery!' And then it goes even further: 'Ben? Take off your trousers, then we can all see your legs better when you're running.'

A few days later, an appointment with the paediatrician: 'Something's not right with Ben's legs – even the teachers at kindergarten have noticed. Get undressed, the doctor wants to examine you. Don't be afraid, it's nothing to worry about!' After the assessment the paediatrician is not sure what to make of it, and says that just to be sure, a child orthopaedist should have a look at Ben. So, on to the child orthopaedist. Here Ben has to take off his trousers and underpants so that the orthopaedist can squeeze cold, slimy gel out of a tube onto his hip, to examine it with an ultrasound device. Ben refuses. Mother:

'Now don't make such a fuss, you aren't going to have an injection, and it won't hurt!' The examination is finally carried out after a fashion, with Ben in tears.

So if a child then comes to Shōnishin for the first time, we can see that he has reason enough to be feeling scared. All too often the child has had to go through the experience of being shown to someone! He simply will not want to be assessed all over again, to have something unpleasant done, yet again – even if it doesn't hurt. But it does hurt if a weakness is repeatedly put on show, and to strangers, above all! For the child there are plenty of reasons not to cooperate.

Therefore, the child is undressed only as far as he will allow. He can sit on his mother's lap and can hide his face against her.

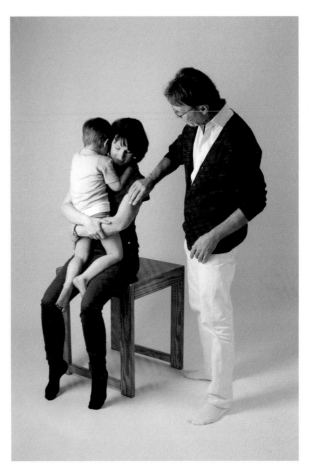

Figure 4.21

The treatment begins with the mother, and in such a way that the child can observe it out of the corner of his eye.

The mother is asked: 'Does this massage feel good?' and she replies, very convincingly: 'Mmm – that's so-oooo good!'

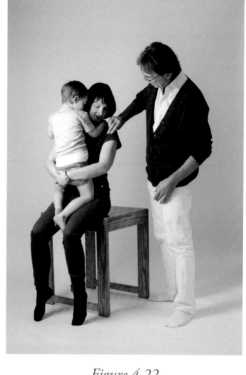

Figure 4.22

As if by chance, you touch the child's forearm. If there is no defensive reaction, you treat him. The child can be expected to 'secretly' watch what is happening. The important thing is to keep up the conversation with the mother throughout the treatment – in this way the contact loses its significance.

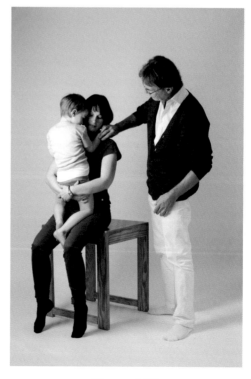

Figure 4.23

Now the child gets curious. So you can 'work your way forward' and make contact with the free hand (Figure 4.24). He even accepts treatment on his back (Figure 4.25) and watches treatment on his leg with interest (Figure 4.26).

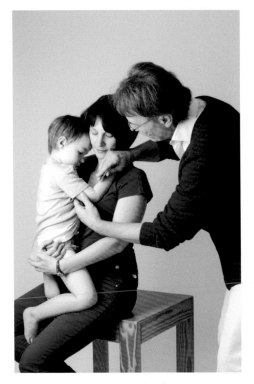

Figure 4.24

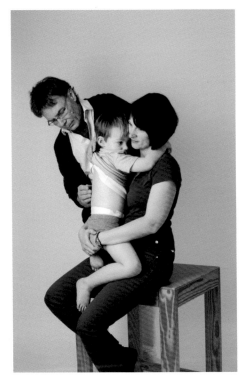

Figure 4.25

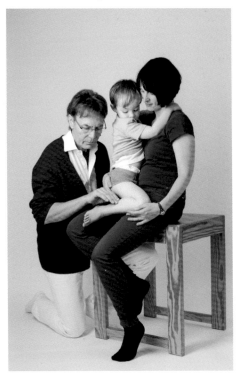

Figure 4.26

The fear has gone. The child is pretty relaxed as tapping treatment is done around the navel (Figure 4.27), and vibration treatment at acupuncture points Lu 9 (Figure 4.28) and Sp 3 can be done without any trouble at all (Figure 4.29).

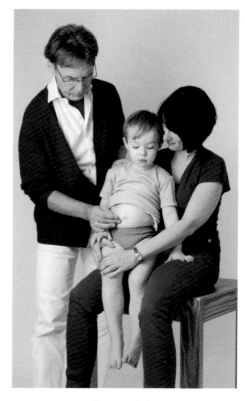

Figure 4.27

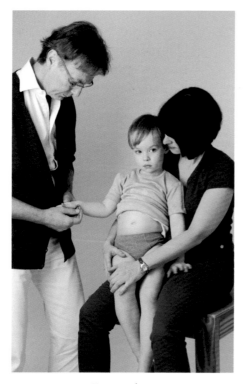

Figure 4.28

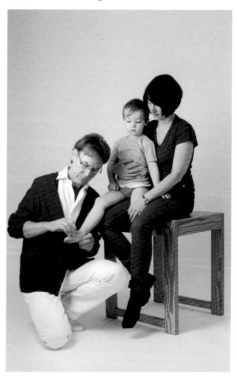

Figure 4.29

4.9 The basic treatment

One of the main pillars of Shōnishin is the basic treatment. This is the foundation of each and every Shōnishin treatment. The basic treatment is always carried out – and that applies to children as well as grown-ups!

From the neurophysiological perspective, we can produce/restore homeostasis by influencing the vegetative nervous system. This comes about thanks to the specific way in which the stroking technique is done in the context of the basic treatment. It creates a state of relaxation in the child, in which the child can self-regulate spontaneously. The child is brought back to, and helped to find, her own centre. With babies the basic treatment can calm excessive dynamics in the *ki*.

The following principle is fundamental in the basic treatment. Work is done:

- predominantly on the domain of the front family

- from cranial to caudal

- from proximal to distal.

This principle corresponds to the sequence in which motor development happens (or has already happened).

This sequence of treatment, shown below in the example of treatment for a baby, has proved to be very effective.

The baby is lying on her back. Before treatment begins, the baby and the practitioner must first have made contact with one another.

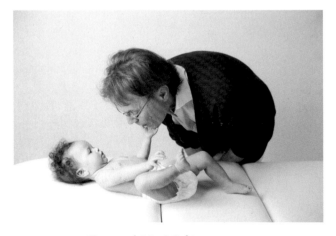

Figure 4.30: Making contact

Begin by stroking the shoulder joint, then continue along the area of what will later be the lung and large intestine meridians on the upper arm and forearm (first one arm, then the other).

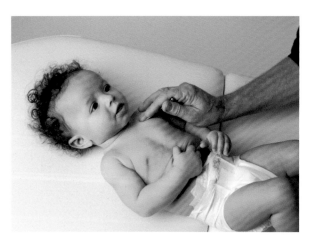

Figure 4.31

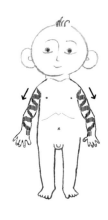

Figure 4.32

Starting from the upper edge of the breastbone (sternum), stroke below the collarbone (clavicle) to the right and left Lung areas (region of Lu 1 and Lu 2)…

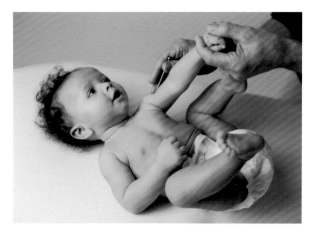

Figure 4.33

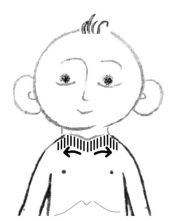

Figure 4.34

...from the upper edge of the sternum down to the xiphoid process (*proc. xiphoideus sterni*)...

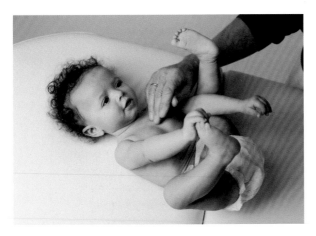

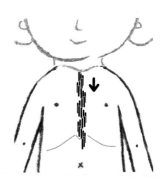

Figure 4.35   *Figure 4.36*

...from there, below the ribcage as far as the right side (and left side respectively) (the region of Li 13)...

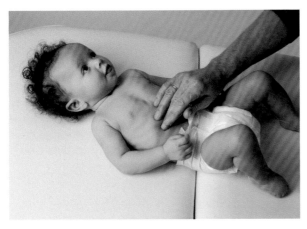

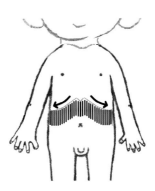

Figure 4.37   *Figure 4.38*

...from the xiphoid process to the navel; clockwise around the navel; from below the navel to the upper edge of the pubic bone...

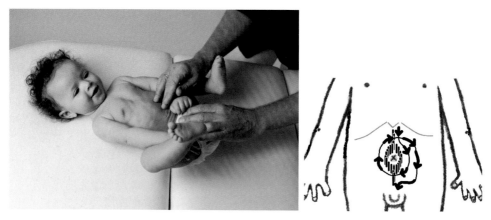

Figure 4.39   Figure 4.40

...from there, across the lumbar area towards the anterior superior iliac spine (*spina iliaca superior anterior*) – first one side, then the other...

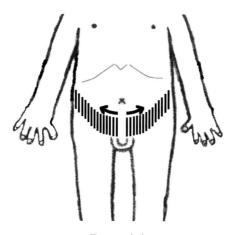

Figure 4.41

…finally, from the hip joint towards the foot along the area of what will later be the stomach and spleen meridians, as far as the ankle (first one leg, then the other).

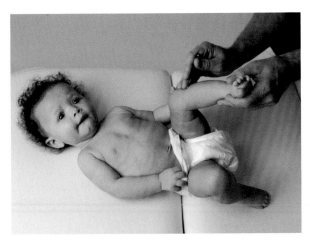

Figure 4.42

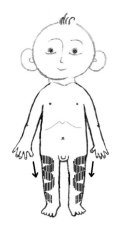

Figure 4.43

Now lay the baby on her front. Stroke from the area of Du Mai 14 on the shoulder, in the direction of the shoulder joint (first one side, then the other)…

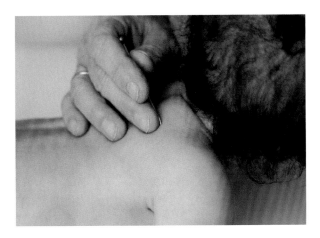

Figure 4.44

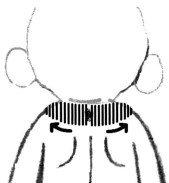

Figure 4.45

... starting from Du Mai, along both sides of the spine down as far as the sacrum...

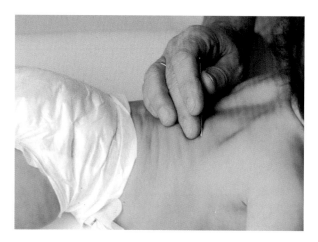

Figure 4.46

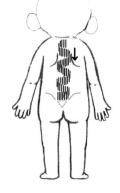

Figure 4.47

...from there, above the crest of the pelvis, outwards towards the right and left sides...

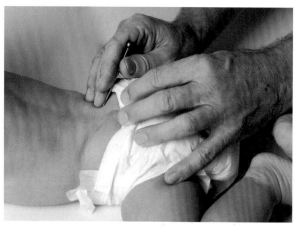

Figure 4.48

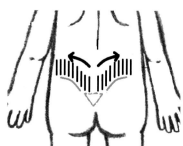

Figure 4.49

...and to finish, over the sacrum towards the tailbone (*coccyx*).

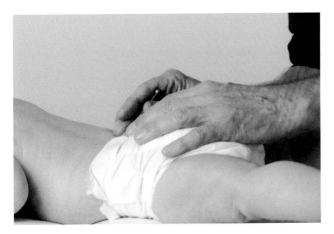

Figure 4.50

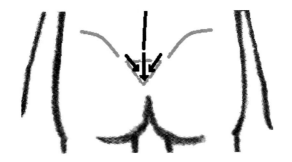

Figure 4.51

With children from the age of about 1 year upwards, a head treatment also forms part of the basic treatment – but not if they are less than 1 year old because of the risk of injury at the anterior fontanelle, which has not yet closed up. Also, babies generally dislike having their heads touched (as parents can confirm when the baby's romper suit is pulled on or off over her head, and the child makes a vociferous protest).

The head treatment is best done with the child sitting, and to best advantage at the end of the basic treatment. Begin at the highest point on the head, which corresponds to the region of Du Mai 20. From there treat the areas of the parietal bone (*os parietale*), the temporal bone (*os temporale*) and the occipital bone (*os occipitale*) with the appropriate stroking technique. No basic treatment is done on the forehead and face.

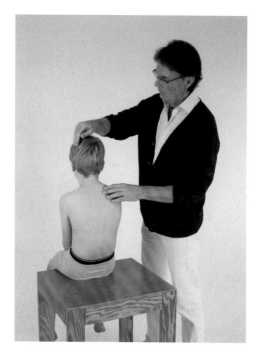

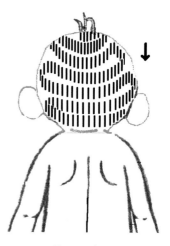

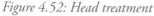

Figure 4.52: Head treatment   *Figure 4.53*

In the following chapter I shall discuss in detail (and following the sequence of the developmental stages) sensorimotor and energetic principles, treatment principles and selected conditions and abnormalities. The patterns of abnormality that are typical for each developmental stage need to be discussed separately for babies, pre-school children and children of school age.

5

Treating Babies
(from Birth to 12 Months)

'Without healthy babies, there are no healthy adults.'
(Shou-chuan *et al.* 2012)

Treating babies presumes knowledge of the special characteristics of babies. Here it is not sufficient to know that children aren't little grown-ups; what is required is more fundamental knowledge about sensorimotor development in infants. Knowing which developmental step is to be expected when in a baby's life, and which not, is of utmost importance in order to carry out treatment with confidence – and deal confidently with the baby's parents. In working to a professional standard, this is key.

5.1 Sensorimotor and energetic principles

Even before birth the baby can already smell, taste and hear. Primitive movement patterns have also been formed, and so the baby can already move her hand to her mouth and suck her thumb. Compared to other mammals, however, the newborn baby is still really undeveloped and completely helpless. Once the umbilical cord has been cut she has to deal with a new, completely unknown situation: she is exposed to the force of gravity, and she feels hungry.

The baby's initially undirected movements ('general movements') become increasingly coordinated. By around three months she has found her centre ('hand-to-hand contact'/'foot-to-foot contact'). By this time she has also learnt to control the position and movement of her head while lying either on her back or on her front ('head control'). At the age of 5 to 6 months she is able to roll from her back onto her tummy, and vice versa. She can't manage to do this until, at some point between the fourth and the sixth month, the structure within the brain that is known as the *corpus callosum* has formed and the two brain hemispheres have connected. Now the baby can reach across the midline of her body and roll over. At 7 to 8 months she can sit unsupported, turn and crawl, until finally at 10 to 12 months the toddler can use objects to pull herself up onto her feet, and then – at last! – at around 13 months she can walk by herself.

See Table 5.1 for a detailed account of the separate stages of sensorimotor development.

Table 5.1: Stages of sensorimotor development during the first 12 months

Age	Sensorimotor development	
	Lying on back	*Lying on front*
1 month	Asymmetrical posture Head turned mostly to one side (but possibly to the other side as well) Aimless movements of arms and legs Hands form slight fists	Lifts head only briefly Able to turn head to both sides Arms bent, lying close to the body Hands forming slight fists Body's centre of gravity: breastbone
6–8 weeks	Begins to lisp, smile Still lying asymmetrically Visual discovery of hands, playing with fingers	First move into upright against gravity – resting on upper arms Shoulder girdle raised off the mattress for the first time Briefly holding head held up (head control) Body's centre of gravity: moving towards the navel
2/3 months	Hands meeting above middle of chest (hand-to-hand contact) Feet touching on the medial side (foot-to-foot contact) Recognises objects within the visual field	

Age	Sensorimotor development	
	Lying on back	*Lying on front*
3/4 months	Spontaneous smiling Beginning to utter sounds Symmetrical posture (with head centred) Raising arms and legs off the mattress Legs bent at 90° at hips and knees, thighs wide apart Lifting bottom slightly off the mattress Head centred, rolling on her own to right and left, without raising her back off the mattress Playing with hands in front of the body, putting hands in mouth Reacting to objects with open hands Following objects with the eyes Targeted reaching for objects; can hold toys placed in hands	Baby lies symmetrically Resting on forearms, with elbows vertically under shoulder joints Holding head up for at least one minute and turning it freely Lower legs raised (to counterbalance the head, which makes up almost one third of body weight) – also bracing the big toes into the mattress Body's centre of gravity: the symphysis
6/7 months	Babbling at toys Holding feet in hands, playing with them, or toes in mouth (hand-to-foot and hand-foot-mouth contact) Able to raise head Hands grabbing at anything within reach, putting it into mouth Arms reaching across centre of the body Actively rolling from back onto front	Raising upper body, supported on both hands Stretching out arms Can lift chest off mattress Body's centre of gravity: thighs Rolling from front onto back (and later from back onto front) Starting to pull herself along

continued

Table 5.1: Stages of sensorimotor development
during the first 12 months *continued*

Age	Sensorimotor development
8/9 months	Afraid of strangers Independent sitting for short periods Pincer grip (grasping with thumb and index finger) Holding bottle by herself Great interest in details and small objects, pointing with index finger at tiny crumbs and picking them up On all fours Beginning to crawl Pulling up into standing position
10–12 months	Crawling all over the place Independent sitting First steps alongside furniture Independent walking for the first time

As explained in detail in section 3.1, energetic development is also incomplete at the time of birth. While it is true that all the main meridians are laid down, more is needed before they can emerge fully. Motor and sensory development helps the rudimentary meridians to develop, while the emerging meridians form the energetic foundation for motor and sensory development. As immature meridians in the groupings known as the 'three families' they generate the principles that are needed for lifelong development: our life themes. They are laid down as resources for us to draw on at any time.

This is an incredible course of development! Parents experience this time as a huge miracle that reveals itself anew every day.

5.2 Principles of treatment

The dynamics of *ki*

Treating babies is very simple. As the separate meridians are still undifferentiated, there is little sense in involving them in treatment. For the most part it's a matter of 'calming' the movement of *ki*, which can be intense during infancy and typically expresses itself in babies with suddenness and vigour.

So in babies a temperature rises not gradually, but all at once, and then significantly. Not only the onset of illness but the healing process also happens a lot faster in babies. So again and again we see an improvement in the presenting condition in the course of a single Shōnishin treatment.

In terms of its quality, *ki* has a yang character (Shou-chuan *et al.* 2012). In children, and in babies especially, the *ki* also tends to shoot upwards, that is, towards the head. Spluttering, hiccups, vomiting, burping, coughing and suddenly crying out are expressions of this upward movement in the flow of *ki*. The *ki* dynamics can very easily throw the baby off centre – therefore this dynamic needs to be regulated.

In paediatrics the most frequent disorders in infancy are called, in neurophysiological terms, 'adjustment disorder' and relate primarily to the subject of 'sleep' and 'digestion'. In the majority of cases adjustment disorder is the result of the vegetative nervous system not yet having come into balance – and this is precisely where the basic treatment begins. But first, before we start on the treatment itself, several conditions need to be met.

Creating a good setting for treatment

The treatment room should be pleasantly warm, or have a commercially available warming lamp for babies positioned directly next to the place where treatment is to be carried out.

In case the young parents have forgotten to bring along a nappy changing mat, a suitable disposable mat should be to hand. It can also be very helpful to have a paper towel within easy reach in case it's necessary to clean up a spluttering baby.

The baby lies on the changing mat, wearing just her nappy. It's advisable to change this before treatment begins, in case the nappy is already wet or soiled – this calms the baby (and the practitioner's sense of smell).

It goes without saying that hands are washed before every treatment – and not with perfumed soap, as more and more babies are allergic to perfume (even natural ones). And be sure that your hands are warm before touching the baby.

Meridian flow and general movements

During the first year of life, usually only the basic treatment is done. Simply regulating the dynamic state of *ki* in the baby can very quickly lead to the disappearance of a range of infantile disorders. In certain areas the vibration technique can be used, especially in the places where the future acupuncture points are forming. This concerns, as a rule, the source points (yuan points) of the developing meridians. Where appropriate, gentle tapping techniques can already be done around the navel, stimulating the area of the spleen functional sphere with the aim of supporting the baby in finding her own centre.

However, at this early developmental stage there is no point in meridian treatment, because so far no directed flow of *ki* has formed within the individual meridians. This can be seen at the motor level from the fact that during the first three to four months the baby consistently demonstrates changing patterns of movement – referred to as 'general movements'. These spontaneous movements are superseded by voluntary movements at the age of 3 to 4 months. Only then is the baby able to carry out targeted movements and reach out for something; and only then is there the beginning of directional flow within the developing meridians. In the insufficiently developed yin meridians the direction of flow is from caudal to cranial, and in the yang meridians from cranial to caudal. The energetic condition for targeted movement has now been met.

By the age of about 1 year sensorimotor development has progressed to the point where the energy is flowing in a directed sequence within the meridians. Only now does it make any sense to do meridian treatment in addition to the basic treatment.

5.3 Conditions and disorders

It is best, of course, if things do not reach the point where children need to be treated. Over 1300 years ago the famous physician Sun Si Miao gave the following advice on how to be healthy in his book *Bei Ji Qian Jin Yao Fang* (*Important Formulas worth a Thousand Gold Pieces for Emergencies*):

> Babies should be brought outside when the weather is pleasant; otherwise, babies are weak and fragile. When it is sunny, warm and not windy, mothers should bring their babies outside to breathe fresh air and bathe in sunshine. Then the babies will be strong and able to defend against wind, cold and disease. (Shou-chuan *et al.* 2012)

Typical disorders that appear in infancy are:

- three-month colic

- KISS syndrome (see section 5.4)

- sleep disturbance

- excessive crying

- vomiting (reflux)

- digestive problems.

Three-month colic

Around 20 per cent of all babies suffer from cramp-like stomach aches in the first months: three-month colic. The precise cause of colic is still unknown, even though many suppositions can be made.

Typically, colic linked with attacks of screaming begins 2 weeks after birth and lasts for about 3 (at most 4) months. It usually begins in the late afternoon and early evening, especially during or soon after a feed. While screaming the baby often writhes with pain, pulling her legs in or arching her body.

Bringing up wind and passing stools can bring relief, and so can light pressure on the abdomen, warmth and being carried around. This distinguishes three-month colic from excessive crying, when nothing has any effect on the baby's screaming. Serious causes of the screaming attacks must also be ruled out. If there is sudden, shrill screaming and, for example, blood in the stools, or a developmental disorder, then a doctor should always be consulted.

SUPPLEMENTARY TREATMENT

- Permanent needle St 25 on both sides (see section 4.4).

  The permanent needle is particularly suitable for use in the treatment of newborns, babies and toddlers. Thanks to its extremely short length the needle cannot penetrate the epidermis, so this is not an invasive technique. This method is even gentler than use of the magnet-plaster or seed-plaster, which, over a few days, can cut into the baby's delicate skin.

  With newborns and babies, digestion is the weak point that is often impossible to miss because of the way the baby screams. In the first months after birth, three-month colic is the main cause of screaming. In this case treatment with the permanent needle is very helpful, as midwives well appreciate.

  The needle can be applied without any problem to left and right of the navel in the area of the developing St 25 acupuncture point (Figure 5.1). Here the needle shows its main strength: thanks to its non-invasive quality, not even the pressure of the nappy on the skin and the warm dampness under it will lead to any irritation in this area. A further advantage of the needles is that bathing and washing won't make the plasters come unstuck.

  Leave the needles in place for three days maximum.

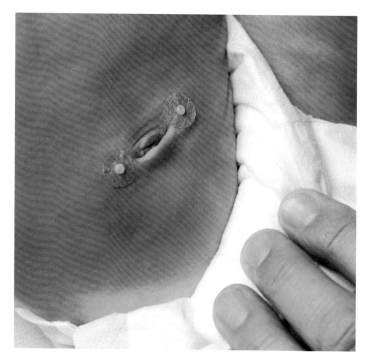

Figure 5.1: Permanent needles at St 25

Tips

- Many babies can be helped if you hold them tightly in your arms or wrap them up tightly in a blanket.

- Many babies are also helped by being carried in the 'flying position'. Take care with this, as the baby will be lying on her tummy on the mother or father's forearm. In this position the pressure on the abdomen makes it easier for air to escape. If the pressure generated by lying on her tummy causes the baby discomfort, you can hold her as shown in Figure 5.2.

- It can help if, with the baby lying on her back, you bend her legs and at the same time the mother or father gently presses a fingertip onto the area of St 36. The painful accumulation of air in the baby's tummy can then escape more easily. Sometimes, this can be achieved simply by laying the baby on her tummy.

- Many babies like skin contact and slow, gentle clockwise stroking on their tummy.

- Others enjoy the weightless feeling of being in a warm bath, which will relax them.

- A change of surroundings, fresh air and a ride in the pram can bring relaxation. Here, however, take care not to create the opposite effect by exposing the child to a constant stream of new stimuli.

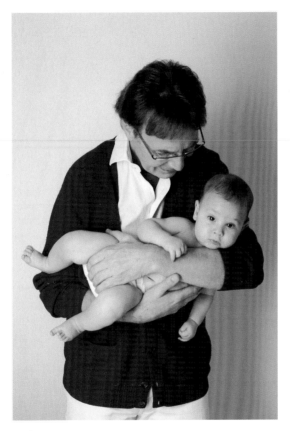

Figure 5.2

Vomiting (reflux)

Many babies are sick ('spitting'/'spluttering'), sometimes copiously, especially after a feed with burping. As long as the baby shows normal weight gain, even if she is sick, there is no cause for concern. But if the baby always vomits copiously and there is concern about weight gain, then it is essential to rule out pyloric stenosis.

SUPPLEMENTARY TREATMENT

- Vibration treatment of the front family source points

- Stroking three times (stroking technique) from the tip of the sternum to the navel (Figure 5.3)

- Vibration treatment (or permanent needle) on Ren 12

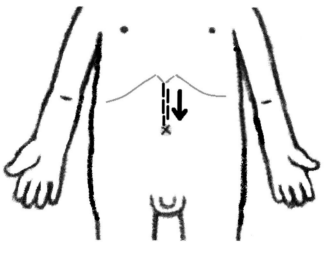

Figure 5.3

Sleep disturbance

For the first few weeks of life babies don't yet have a sleep rhythm that could be disturbed. Sixteen to eighteen hours' sleep means that the short spells when they are awake are filled by the feeds that are necessary up to 10 times daily, and nappy changes. Only gradually do they develop a rhythm. So here we are not yet talking of sleep disturbance.

Nevertheless, we often see a baby that has scarcely fallen asleep before she wakes up screaming. This may be the 'fault' of the Moro reflex, which can be set off by, amongst other things, noises, startling events and the transition between different phases of sleep. Here the following sequence can be observed:

- The baby opens her eyes and mouth wide; the arms move jerkily outwards with the fingers spread wide, hitting the mattress.

- The baby's mouth shuts and the arms return to the sides of the body.

- Then, in many cases, the baby screams.

Many babies are awoken by the sudden and unintentional twitching and react with attacks of crying. After the third or fourth month the Moro reflex gradually disappears, and with it the sleep disturbance that it creates.

Another cause of babies sleeping badly or having problems falling asleep is an increasing restlessness that comes over them as evening approaches. Their eyes redden and they start to whimper more and more, which can rapidly progress to crying. It is not uncommon for them to take hours to fall asleep – a nervous ordeal for the parents and the child.

Supplementary treatment

- Vibration treatment; when appropriate, permanent needle at Bl 15, St 25 or Ren 12 (depending on the cause).

Tips

- As many parents believe that it's easier for their baby to fall asleep when she's really tired, they often make the mistake of putting their child to bed as late as possible. Unfortunately, the effect is exactly the opposite of what the parents hoped for – their baby is now overwrought, can't settle down, and when she does finally fall asleep, it's not the deep sleep that is needed for recovery.

- Plan sufficient time for the going-to-bed ritual.

- If the baby wakes up in the night, keep it simple: giving her a drink, breastfeeding and nappy changing can all be done without much light and without a lot of talking.

- If the baby awakes because of a Moro reflex that is easily set off, swaddling may help. Swaddling is a special way of wrapping a baby that makes falling asleep and sleeping through easier for them. It gives them a special feeling of warmth, peace and security – similar to the safe feeling inside the womb. Because a swaddled baby's arms can't twitch uncontrollably, she won't be rudely awakened (and kept awake) by this.

- See Chapter 11 on treatment at home.

- 'Clasp your child's ankles, and with your thumbs apply a little pressure to the hollow in the soles of both feet for a minute or two. This point is called "Bubbling Spring". Touching this point calms the baby and helps it sleep' (Kalbantner-Wernicke 2010).

Excessive crying

Of course, there are always times when all is not a bed of roses – for example, when the baby is crying. There are days when she just won't calm down, and all attempts to make her feel better come to nothing. She may be hungry, sore, bored, or just wants Mummy – there are any number of reasons.

Visitors can also be a challenge. Friends and relations want to see the new member of the family and give her presents and a cuddle. For the baby this means being constantly exposed to strange people, strange voices and strange smells. She's always being picked up by another person she doesn't know. Pretty stressful for the baby, and sometimes, indeed, quite a burden! Newborns especially are quickly overwhelmed in these situations.

On top of this, at around six weeks the baby loses her defence against stimuli that protected her from being inundated with sensory impressions in the first weeks following birth, rather like an invisible wall. Now all the stimuli that she was previously able to shut out stream in on her without let or hindrance. Therefore, in the early days, babies cry more to get rid of the tension that has built up. This usually happens in the afternoon or evening, when the strain has accumulated over the course of the day.

However, this has nothing to do with excessive crying. According to American paediatrician Morris Wessel's 1954 definition, which is still accurate today, we can talk of excessive crying if the 'rule of threes' is met. This rule states that the screaming has to occur for over three hours a day, on at least three days a week, for a spell of at least three weeks. This much is certain: a lot of young parents faced with excessive crying would be glad if this were true of their baby. It can be quite different: 60 to 120 minutes uninterrupted crying, then 20 minutes dozing with exhaustion, then crying again for up to two hours – doze, cry, etc. – for 24 hours a day.

For the parents this means sleep deprivation. Only those who have experienced something of the sort know how cruel it can be – it's like torture. Parents affected by it may reach a state of diminished responsibility – we are dealing here with an emergency! Waiting, letting it carry on, can have unforeseen consequences – with a excessive crying there has to be prompt action.

> It is the implacable nature of the attacks of screaming, the crying for no identifiable reason, and the long phases of inexplicable restlessness and whimpering, that are characteristic of excessive crying. (Ziegler, Wollwerth and Papousek, in Papusek *et al.* 2004)

The causes of these screaming attacks can be very different:

- Gastroenterological disorder/illness, such as:

  - intolerance of the protein in cows' milk (5–10% of all babies with excessive crying)

  - gastro-oesophageal reflux (max. 5% of all babies with excessive crying).

- KISS syndrome (60% (Biedermann 2000) and, in our own experience, around 80% of all babies with excessive crying).

SUPPLEMENTARY TREATMENT

- Where appropriate, permanent needle at Bl 15, St 25, Ren 12 (depending on the cause).

Tips

- The baby has to be protected from overstimulation – she can't defend herself! So don't feel guilty if this means declining a visit from somebody.

- If visitors come to the door unannounced, or your mobile rings just as you are breastfeeding or giving the baby the bottle, you don't have to open the door or answer the call. More important is to have the peace and quiet that mother and baby need. The visitor can try again another day.

- If the baby is crying, don't try to distract her – with a rattle, for example. As a rule, this will make the crying and screaming worse. Instead, it's better to go to a quiet place such as a darkened room. As many babies strongly desire the mother's proximity and body contact at this age, what frequently helps the most is simply holding the baby in your arms as a way of showing her that someone is there for her.

Digestive problems

DIARRHOEA

With diarrhoea there is frequent, sometimes explosive voiding of loose or watery stools. In babies diarrhoea, like vomiting, carries the risk of dehydration. Therefore the most important thing is to ensure sufficient liquid and mineral intake.

Not every loose stool is diarrhoea; especially in babies who are breastfed, a thin, yellow stool passed several times a day is completely normal.

Supplementary treatment

- Vibration treatment of front family source points

- Permanent needles in the region of St 25 (on both sides)

- Gentle tapping treatment around the navel – anti-clockwise (Figure 5.4)

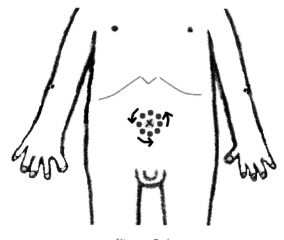

Figure 5.4

- Tapping treatment above the rim of the pelvis – from the inside outwards (Figure 5.5)

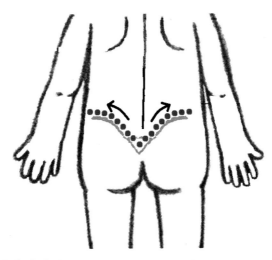

Figure 5.5

Tip

- With fingertips or the flat of the hand, stroke (don't massage!) slowly and gently anti-clockwise around the navel.

CONSTIPATION

Unweaned children can pass stools up to seven times a day, and older children twice a day. In unweaned children there may be no bowel movement for as long as 10 days. This is only a question of constipation if opening the bowels is delayed for longer than usual, or if stools that are too infrequent or too hard are causing difficulties.

There is nothing the matter if weaning (changing the infant over from breast milk to other food) causes constipation in the short term. Basically this is no cause for concern as long as the child shows no sign of discomfort. On the other hand, if there is persistent crying, vomiting or blood in the nappy, a doctor should be consulted at once – and the same if the newborn has not passed a stool within the first few days after birth, as this may be a sign of a more serious illness, such as cystic fibrosis, Hirschsprung's disease, underactive thyroid or malformation of the intestine.

Supplementary treatment

- Vibration treatment of front family source points

- Vibration treatment of the St 25 region, on both sides

- Gentle tapping treatment around the navel, clockwise (Figure 5.6)

- Tapping treatment above the rim of the pelvis, starting from the lateral side: from the outside inwards (Figure 5.7)

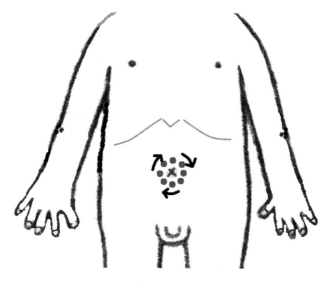

Figure 5.6

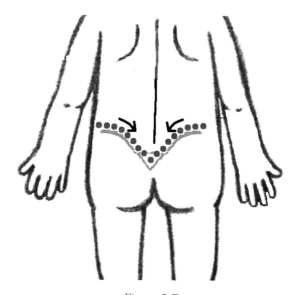

Figure 5.7

Tips

- With fingertips or the flat of the hand, stroke (don't massage!) slowly and gently clockwise around the navel.

- Massage the point called 'Divine Equanimity' below and to one side of the baby's knee. You can find it by sliding your thumb gently upwards between the tibia and fibula, stopping a finger's breadth below the kneecap. Hold the point for about one minute, following the baby's kicking movements (Kalbantner-Wernicke 2010).

5.4 KISS babies

KISS syndrome

The first three months are decisive in a baby's development. During this time the course of further development is set. The capabilities the baby gains during this time will continue for life. This also applies to capabilities that are wrongly programmed – correcting these subsequently is a laborious and sometimes frustrating enterprise. Therefore the first three months of a baby's life are really important.

This is also the reason why treatment of babies with KISS syndrome is best done between the sixth and twelfth weeks of life. An understanding of the most important developmental steps during this time is also needed. For good measure, these are summarised in Table 5.2.

The degree to which sensorimotor and energetic development are interlinked has already been explained (see section 3.1). From this we can see how, according to the theory of energetic development, the meridians are a communication network between the child's developing consciousness and the external world. They are equally responsible for the integration of reflexes and stimuli, and the development of a child's posture, movement and patterns of personality and behaviour.

How sensitive the interplay within the communication network is can be seen from the multitude of abnormalities that can arise if there are any disturbances, and which may be expressed, for example, as difficulties in bonding, disturbances in perception, motor abnormalities, or delayed development to the point of developmental disorder. In KISS syndrome the variety of abnormalities is strikingly evident. Here a localised abnormality in the cervical spine exerts such an influence on the sensitive system of sensorimotor and energetic linkage that this one abnormality can in itself produce a whole range of widely different symptoms.

Table 5.2: Developmental stages during weeks 6 to 12

Age	Lying on back	Lying on front
6–8 weeks	Unstable when lying Finding centre of body for the first time (HHC) Visual discovery of hands; playing with fingers Recognising objects in visual field Beginning to lisp, smile	Leaning on forearms Brief control of head Lifting shoulder girdle off mattress for the first time Centre of gravity: the navel
9–12 weeks	Symmetrical posture (head centred) Raising arms and legs Head centred, turning to right and left Hands touching over middle of chest; looking at hands Reaching out for objects Feet meeting Smiling spontaneously	Leaning on elbows Holding head up for at least one minute and turning it freely Child should be symmetrical Centre of gravity: moving towards the symphase

DEFINITION OF KISS

As early as the 1970s and 1980s, random examinations of newborn babies (Seifert 1975; Buchmann and Bülow 1983) showed (according to different authors) that some 27–33 per cent of all babies had movement disorders resulting from a segmental dysfunction (often called a 'blockage') of the suboccipital joints. What they were talking about is 'KISS syndrome'.

The term KISS (Kinematic Imbalances due to Suboccipital Strain) was first used by children's orthopaedist Dr Biedermann (1991) and applies to babies and toddlers. The term encapsulates what we know about the cause of asymmetrical babies and toddlers, whose appearance is striking, in particular because of the crooked head position and scoliotic posture of the trunk, in addition to disorders in vegetative functions. As the term KISS implies, it concerns a disorder the cause of which is to be found in the area of the suboccipital joints (Figure 5.8).

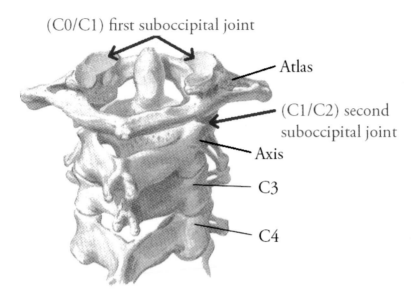

(C0/C1) first suboccipital joint

Atlas

(C1/C2) second suboccipital joint

Axis

C3

C4

Figure 5.8: The suboccipital joints

The importance of the suboccipital joints

That the asymmetry stems, in most cases, from a blockage is evident from the fact that, as a rule, it is quickly reversed once the blockage has been removed. The role of the suboccipital joints here derives from the fact that the suboccipital joints and the structures in this area form a sensory organ and are of critical importance in the transition to the human upright posture, from four legs to two.

How is it that the suboccipital joints play such an important part? The upper cervical region (comprising) the suboccipital joints especially is characterised by a very high concentration of receptors. For example, the density of muscle spindles in the short neck muscles in that area is twice that in the muscles of the hand. Receptors for proprioception, motor control and pain processing (nociception) are concentrated in this area.

This explains the importance of this receptor field for the development of posture and balance. And it explains the body's instant reaction to faulty information. All this is especially applicable to babies and toddlers. As a result, unilateral malfunctions of the suboccipital joints lead to asymmetrical control of muscular tonus (Biedermann 2000), which in turn leads to higher muscle tension on one side of the body compared to the other – hence the 'crooked baby'.

The impact of childbirth on the suboccipital joints

In most cases the cause of asymmetry is to be found in the birthing process. That said, it appears not to be important whether the delivery took place naturally, with forceps or by Caesarean section; there are always more or less strong forces of compression and traction on the cervical spine in particular, mostly linked with torsion, flexion and hyperextension in this area. Especially if there is a hiatus in the birth process and rapid measures need to be taken (forceps, suction cup, external pressure applied to the mother's abdomen), this increases the risk of a blockage in the suboccipital joints. Additional risk factors for asymmetry are, among others: multiple pregnancy, baby in the wrong position in the womb, pre-term births, precipitate delivery, oxytocia (Sacher 2006).

Symptoms

The principal symptom is fixed posture, caused in most cases by birth trauma irritating the upper cervical spine. This leads to permanent and painful restriction of movement in the head–neck region. Abnormalities in this area often have an impact on almost all areas of the body and their functions.

Segment C1/C2

Depending which is the affected segment in the cervical spine, different postures result (Biedermann 1991). If a blockage between the atlas (C1) and the axis (C2) is the cause of restricted movement, then the head is rotated to one side, with a sideways tilt towards the opposite side – this is called 'KISS I'.

Segment C0/C1

In KISS II we find the movement restriction one segment higher up, between the occiput (C0) and the atlas (C1). A blockage in this segment can be recognised by fixed retroflexion of the head with hyperextension of the entire trunk. KISS I and KISS II rarely present in their pure form – usually there is a combination of the two basic forms.

You only have to look more closely at a baby in order to recognise the indicators of KISS. If you know what to look for, the signs are not difficult to recognise. All the symptoms listed in Table 5.3 can appear separately. The more symptoms that are visible, the more likely it is that KISS syndrome is present.

Table 5.3: Symptoms and abnormalities in KISS syndrome

Physical symptoms and abnormalities
Skewed position of head
Can't hold head up
Hyper-extension
Dislikes lying on front
Difficulty crawling
Deformity of the head
Eye open wider on one side
Hands/feet are damp, cold
Developmental delay
Excessive crying
Breastfeeding problems, drooling
Sleep disturbance
Crying in sleep

Vegetative symptoms

There is also a range of signs that indicate KISS syndrome for those who are not familiar with manual examination techniques. Top of the list are vegetative symptoms, which can be explained as follows.

Owing to the direct proximity of some of the 12 cranial nerves, and more especially the proximity of the vegetative nervous system (*ganglion cervicalis superius*) to the upper cervical spine (Figure 5.9), a blockage in the suboccipital joints will lead to increased tonus of the tissue structures located in this area. This in turn leads, in many cases, to irritation of the sympathetic spinal cord in the upper cervical spine, with the result that peripheral organs are also exposed to the effects of stress on the sympathetic nervous system (Kuklinski 2007).

This is the reason for the range of symptoms that may present if there is a blockage in the suboccipital joints (Table 5.4).

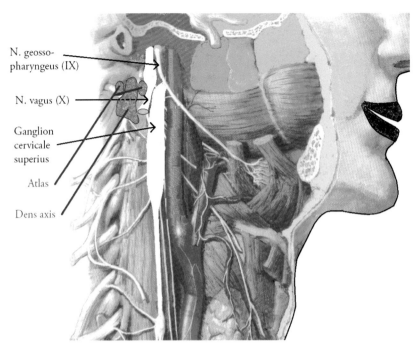

N. geosso-
pharyngeus (IX)

N. vagus (X)

Ganglion
cervicale
superius

Atlas

Dens axis

*Figure 5.9: Spatial proximity of cranial nerves and the vegetative
nervous system in the region of the suboccipital joints*
Note: (IX) and (X) above denote the ninth and tenth cranial nerves.

Table 5.4: Typical symptoms associated with cases of blockage in the suboccipital joints

Additional characteristics caused by irritation of the vegetative nervous system (stimulation of the sympathetic NS)	Additional characteristics caused by irritation of cranial nerve (appropriate cranial nerve given in roman numerals)
Increased muscle tone (hyperextension of the trunk; making fists more often) Damp, cold hands and feet Excessive crying Sleep disturbance Fearful Withholding stools; diarrhoea Facial pallor	Sensitivity to noise (VIII) Resists change of lying position (VIII) Difficulty breastfeeding/taking the bottle owing to hypersensivity of mouth/pharynx (IX) Tendency to diarrhoea (X) Restlessness (X) Weak sucking (XII)

It is important to be aware that all these symptoms do not necessarily point to KISS syndrome. They can also appear when there is no underlying pathology. However, this is not often the case. Other causes that can occur (but fortunately only rarely) are, for example, meningitis, tumour, cerebral palsy or degenerative muscle diseases, which have similar or identical symptoms.

Consequence of failure to treat KISS in a baby

There is no reason to stir up anxiety here, as an untreated KISS baby can appear completely normal in later life. But it turns out that there is an increased probability of untreated KISS babies having various disorders later on. Many indicators of KISS syndrome that was not recognised or treated in infancy are listed (with reference to children aged 4–13) in Table 5.5.

Table 5.5: Indicators of untreated KISS syndrome in children aged 4–13

Late consequences of KISS
Developmental delay
Poor gross and/or fine motor skills
Motor restlessness
Hyperactivity
Poor concentration
Delayed speech and language development
Postural weakness or postural defects
Headache
Recurrent inflammation of the middle ear
Proprioceptive disorder
Clumsiness
Uneven gait
Disorders of sensorimotor processing (auditory, visual, kinaesthetic)

In adulthood, untreated KISS syndrome can lead to a range of problems that are avoidable if treated in time – for example, migraine, headache, tinnitus, vertigo, transient visual disturbance, sinusitis, back pain and digestive problems.

As with KISS symptoms in early childhood, so too with 4–13-year-olds and adults: untreated KISS syndrome does not necessarily underlie the presenting symptoms. However, the spine does play a predominant role in most cases, so once other causes have been ruled out one should always consider a functional disorder of the suboccipital joints.

The variety and intensity of symptoms of KISS syndrome indicate that:

- It is not acceptable to wait for a spontaneous cure, particularly because the longer abnormal postural and behavioural patterns continue, the harder it is to change them.

- Late consequences can be avoided with early treatment, and for this reason non-treatment must be regarded as irresponsible.

Shōnishin: a clinical study

I have been treating babies with KISS for over 20 years, using manual therapeutic and osteopathic/cranio-sacral treatment methods in combination with Shōnishin. Again and again I have seen the blockage in the area of the suboccipital joints disappear as a result of Shōnishin alone (i.e. without manual intervention).

So I asked myself whether these blockages disappearing after Shōnishin were exceptional cases, or whether they could be reproduced. If the latter proved to be the case, then, using Shōnishin as the sole method of treatment, it would be interesting to know the probability for successful removal of a blockage in the suboccipital area, and hence the reduction of associated symptoms that were mostly vegetative in origin (see Table 5.4).

I set myself the task of doing a clinical study to shed light on this question in accordance with scientific criteria. Based exclusively on Shōnishin treatment, I wanted to establish the efficacy of this method in working with babies with KISS. Proof of efficacy was to be demonstrated by the following effects of treatment:

- removal of blockage/s in the region of the suboccipital joints

- improvement in/disappearance of asymmetry

- improvement in associated symptoms.

A further aim of the study was to establish Shōnishin as an effective treatment method – pleasant for the baby and cost-effective for the parents.

My chief motivation for carrying out the study was that demonstrably successful treatment by means of Shōnishin alone would doubtless be of interest for future treatment of babies with KISS syndrome, as the treatment is free of side effects, pleasant, and differs from other treatment methods in the short course of therapy (at most, three sessions) and short duration of individual treatments (around three to five minutes). In addition, Shōnishin has the advantage that it can be done with restless and even crying babies – a situation in which manual therapy, osteopathy or cranio-sacral work is either limited or cannot be done at all.

Implementing the study

The study took place at *therapeuticum rhein-main* with cooperation from four paediatricians from the Rhein-Main region. There has been close collaboration between *therapeuticum rhein-main* and these paediatricians for many years. Regular referrals were (and are) made for diagnosis and/or treatment – with preference given to asymmetrical babies, and toddlers, 4–13-year-olds with behavioural or motor abnormalities.

The babies the paediatricians put forward for this study were within the framework of the 'U3' (a medical check in Germany for babies aged 4–6 weeks) on account of their asymmetry. Of these asymmetrical babies the ones selected for the study were only those with asymmetry caused exclusively by a blockage in the suboccipital joints.

Forty babies who met the following selection criteria were accepted into the study:

- age not less than 6 weeks and not more than 12 weeks

- presenting with KISS syndrome

- no other treatment permitted over the three-week treatment and observation period, in particular no manual therapy, physiotherapy, osteopathy or cranio-sacral work.

Treatment given was exclusively Shōnishin, following a standardised plan. Each baby received three treatments, once a week, at weekly intervals. Each treatment lasted about three to five minutes.

At the start of a course of treatment and one week after the last treatment a manual, full-body diagnostic examination was done and photographically documented (Figure 5.10), paying particular attention to the suboccipital joints. For this, collaboration was required on the part of the mothers (or fathers), using a rattle (occasionally, with boys, it had to be a mobile phone) to get their babies to move their heads in various directions.

The time frame for the study was planned so as to allow time not only for manual therapy treatment, but also for other therapies (e.g. physiotherapy, baby Shiatsu, osteopathy) if required. On ethical grounds, there was no control group.

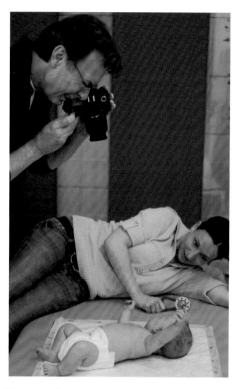

Figure 5.10: Photographic documentation of active rotation of the head

TREATMENT

All the babies were treated according to the same procedure:

- Basic treatment.

- Vibration treatment:

  - The acupuncture points were chosen to address the basic problem in infant asymmetry: absence of the centre – since at the age of 12 weeks hand–hand/foot–foot contact should have happened, enabling the baby to find her centre. The developing meridians that are responsible for the 'centre' receive an impulse for development through stimulation by vibration of the yuan points of the front family (with one exception, St 36, which has proved to be more effective than St 42).

  - In order to achieve rotation of the head while lying in the prone position (this is a function of the developing gallbladder meridian), it is necessary to be able to raise the head, as well as rotate the cervical spine freely (a function of the bladder and small intestine meridians).

If there is a blockage, the potential for doing these movements (raising and rotating the head) has to be activated.

- Tapping treatment on selected areas:

  - In order to obtain further accentuation of the 'centre', tapping treatment is done around the navel (periumbilical), corresponding to the spleen area of the *hara* zone.

  - Next there is a tapping treatment along the developing bladder meridian in order to provoke a reflex response (the infantile Galant reaction) that leads to shortening of the trunk on one side with simultaneous lengthening on the opposite side, thereby stimulating the developing gallbladder meridian. Activating the bladder and gallbladder meridians leads in turn to stimulation of the acupuncture points that are important for rotation of the cervical spine (Bl 10 and Gb 20).

Summary of Shōnishin treatment techniques and their effects

Basic treatment (Figures 5.11 and 5.12)	To regulate *ki*
Vibration treatment Lu 9, LI 4 (Figures 5.13 and 5.14), St 36, Sp 3	To emphasise the centre (an essential precondition for symmetry)
SI 3	Because of its close connection with the cervical spine
Li 3 (Figure 5.15)	To lower generally increased muscle tone
Du Mai 14	To relax the shoulder girdle
SI 9	Because of its close connection with the shoulder blade
Bl 28	Because of its close connection with the sacro-iliac joint

Bl 60 (Figure 5.16)	Because of its effect conducive to becoming upright (leads to better head control in the frontal lying position)
Periumbilical tapping treatment (Figure 5.17)	To emphasise the centre
Tapping treatment on the maturing bladder meridian at the level of the scapulae (Figures 5.18–5.20) or in the lumbar region	To stimulate the gallbladder meridian (necessary for ability to rotate the spine) by provoking a Galant reaction

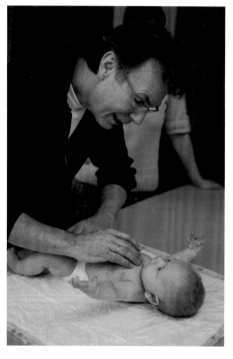

Figure 5.11: Basic treatment in the thoracic area

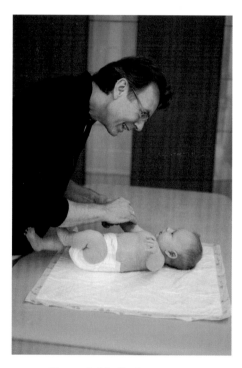

Figure 5.12: Basic treatment on the extremities

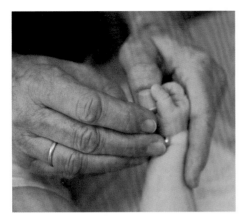

Figure 5.13: Lu 9

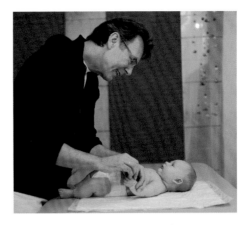

Figure 5.14: LI 4

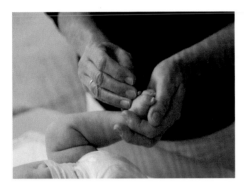

Figure 5.15: Li 3

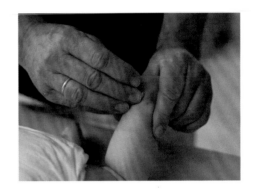

Figure 5.16: Bl 60

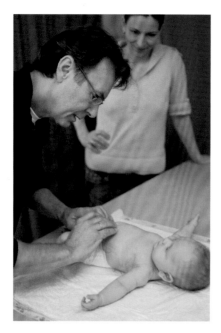

*Figure 5.17: Periumbilical
tapping treatment*

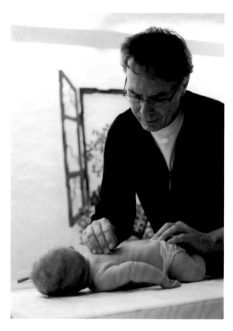

*Figure 5.18: Tapping treatment on bladder
meridian (at the level of the scapulae)*

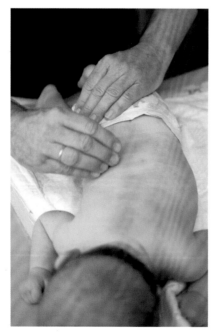

*Figure 5.19: Lateral flexion on the
right side with simultaneous extension
on the contralateral side of the trunk*

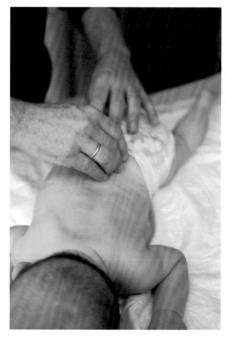

*Figure 5.20: Lateral flexion on the left
side with simultaneous extension on
the contralateral side of the trunk*

ASSESSMENT

A week before the first treatment and a week after the third treatment, each baby was examined on specific (functional–diagnostic) criteria, involving assessment of:

- muscle tone (Figure 5.21) (normal? hypertonic? hypotonic?)

- position of the head (consistently to one side?)

- segmental blockage (visual diagnosis of posture and movement control, careful palpation in the region of the cervical spine)

- position of the trunk (Figure 5.22) (distinctly asymmetrical on one side?)

- form of the face (Figure 5.23) (facial scoliosis and/or deformity of facial bones?)

- eyelids (narrowed on one side?)

- posture and movement pattern of the extremities (abnormal, especially one-sided movement pattern of the extremities and unusual positions of the arms and legs?)

- forming a fist (increased? thumb on the inside?)

- temperature and moisture on the palms of the hands and soles of the feet (caused by irritation of the vegetative nervous system)

- pelvis/sacroiliac joint/position of the feet (blockages of the sacroiliac joints (Buchmann 1983) and position of the feet (Coenen 2011) are described in the literature as frequent adjuncts to a blockage in the suboccipital region)

- form of the head (Figures 5.24a and 5.24b) (holding the head to one side usually leads to flattening of the back of the head on the side it rests on when lying down)

- head control (from the sixth week, fleeting raising of the head while in the prone lying position; from the ninth week, holding the head up for at least one minute)

- using forearms for support (resting on the forearms from the sixth week, and on the elbows from the ninth week).

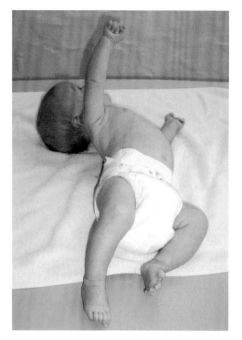

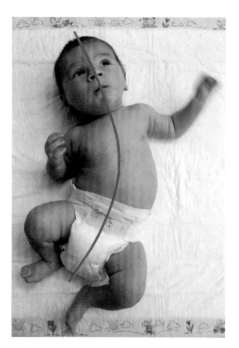

Figure 5.21: Hypertonic muscle tension with overextension

Figure 5.22: Trunk posture convex towards the left

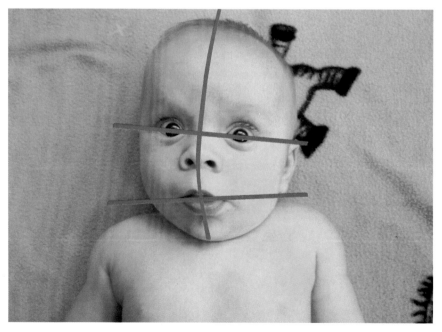

Figure 5.23: Face convex to the right with flattening of the left side of the forehead and left cheek (deviation of the axis of the face shown in red)

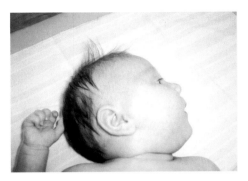 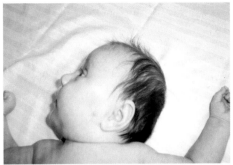

Figure 5.24a: Turning the head…   *Figure 5.24b: …to the right reveals back of the head flattened on the left side*

Results

The following results relate to:

- functionality of the suboccipital joints

- postural and movement patterns

- level of sensorimotor development

- regulation of the vegetative system (its ability to keep vital functions under control).

Functionality of the suboccipital joints

The babies were assessed for evidence of a blockage in the suboccipital area. The results were as follows.

In 23 (57.5%) of the 40 babies there was no longer any sign of the blockage pattern after three Shōnishin treatments (i.e. the segmental dysfunction could be successfully treated by means of Shōnishin alone).

More detailed examination of the remaining 17 babies with persisting suboccipital blockage showed the following distribution:

- In 13 babies (32.5%) there was residual blockage with restricted functionality of 5 degrees on one side compared to the other. Three more babies had restricted functionality of up to 10 degrees, and in one baby the restriction was over 10 degrees.

- Of these 17 babies, 13 were treated with manual therapy. Four of the babies with a 5-degree restriction were not treated, because following successful examination the residual asymmetry in these babies had already disappeared.

Postural and movement patterns

Head position

In order to assess postural patterns, we referred to the positions of the head and trunk in particular. With regard to the head position, only 13 (32.5%) of the 40 babies still had lateral inclination of the head post-treatment, compared to 38 babies (95%) pre-treatment (Figures 5.25a and 5.25b).

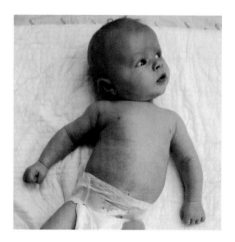

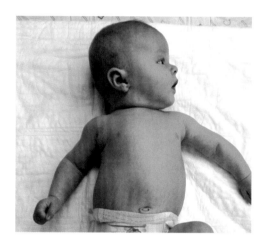

Figure 5.25a: When looking in the direction of the blockage the head is rotated to the left with inclination to the right (before the first treatment)

Figure 5.25b: After the third treatment, the head rotates freely, without lateral inclination

Trunk position

Results of treatment were similarly positive with regard to trunk position (Figures 5.26a–5.26d). Whereas pre-treatment only 10 babies (25%) had symmetrical posture of the trunk, the number of symmetrical babies increased to 33 (82.5%).

Regulation of the vegetative system

In the pre-/post-questionnaires the parents had evaluated 24 symptoms in their babies, as they perceived them both before and on completion of treatment. The six most evident improvements related to the symptoms in Table 5.7.

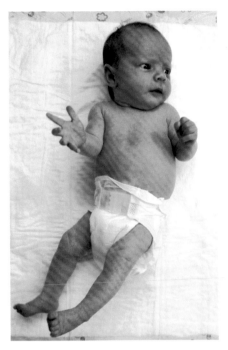

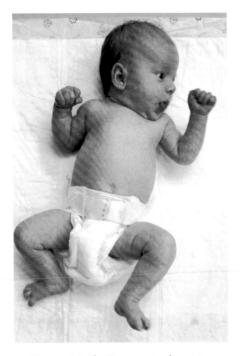

Figure 5.26a: Head rotated in the direction of the blockage – left-convex scoliosis (before the first treatment)

Figure 5.26b: Symmetrical position (after the third treatment)

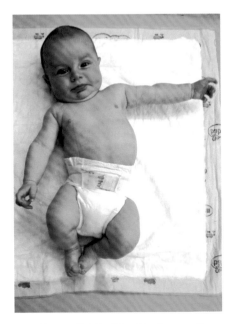

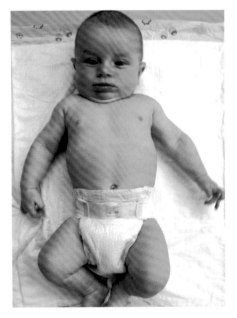

Figure 5.26c: Head in 'neutral' position – left-convex scoliosis (before the first treatment)

Figure 5.26d: Symmetrical position (after the third treatment)

Table 5.7: The most pronounced symptomatic improvements

The most pronounced symptomatic improvements were in:	No. of babies with improvement in symptoms (out of 40)	%
Low tolerance of prone lying position	29	72.5
Recurrent crying	28	70.0
Poor sleep	25	62.5
Recurrent bloating	25	62.5
High degree of restlessness and imbalance	22	55.0
Increased sensitivity to touch on the head	22	55.0

Further treatment

Taking the presenting criteria into account (functionality of the suboccipital joints, posture and movement patterns, sensorimotor state of development, regulation of the vegetative system), it was decided whether further treatment by one of the following interventions was indicated:

- manual therapy

- physiotherapy or baby Shiatsu

- manual therapy combined with physiotherapy.

So 24 babies (and another seven babies in whom it was possible to release the blockage) received additional treatment (physiotherapy/baby Shiatsu) because they were not yet able to carry out their movement and/or postural patterns correctly. In particular, head control and leaning on the elbows showed no clear improvement, despite successful treatment of blockages in the area of the suboccipital joints.

From this we can see that successful treatment of a blockage, even when it removes the asymmetry, does not necessarily mean that a baby gains access to its physiological movement patterns. Whatever movement patterns it hasn't learned in the first 6–12 weeks cannot be anchored in the brain within this time.

In order to encourage sensorimotor development it is important to remove the cause of KISS syndrome (Kalbantner-Wernicke and Wernicke 2010). Only free mobility, of the suboccipital joints in particular, allows physiological programming of movement patterns, and thereby age-appropriate sensorimotor development.

Parental judgement

The parents also had a say. Besides being asked for their assessment of symptoms improved by Shōnishin treatment, parents were also asked about successful/unsuccessful treatment with Shōnishin, and about their satisfaction/dissatisfaction with treatment.

On the question of how they evaluated the success of Shōnishin treatment for their child, 72.5 per cent rated the treatment as very successful or successful, 25 per cent saw a slight improvement, and the treatment was only once rated as unsuccessful.

On the question of satisfaction with treatment, 77.5 per cent of parents were very satisfied or satisfied; 22.5 per cent of those questioned were undecided. None was dissatisfied with the treatment.

Under 'We particularly liked…' the parents could comment freely on anything within the remit of the treatment. In summary, 12 of the 25 parents described Shōnishin as a gentle method ('gentle', 'delicate and enjoyable for our child', 'painless'); nine parents found the treatment relaxing for their child ('completely stress-free', 'calm and alert during treatment', 'expresses wellbeing', 'our child seems to like the method') and four were impressed by how little effort Shōnishin involved ('produced improvement with very little effort', 'it took so little to achieve so much').

Summary

Shōnishin's efficacy is suggested by the following results of treatment:

- In 23 (around 58%) of all the babies treated, release of blockage/s in the area of the suboccipital joints was achieved by treatment with Shōnishin alone.

- Disappearance of asymmetry could be demonstrated in 17 (around 43%) of all the asymmetrical babies treated.

- Many accompanying symptoms showed a clear tendency to improve. In particular, this was true for acceptance of the prone lying position, and behaviours linked with crying and with sleep.

6

Treating Toddlers

The term 'toddler' identifies the life phase comprising the second and third years of life. It is a time of transition in which 'four-legs' is converted to two.

6.1 Sensorimotor and energetic principles

Shuffling and crawling are in the past. Now it's time for walking. Sitting, crawling, standing, taking a few steps, stumbling, and down into a squat – the toddler's posture and body position are changing all the time. Walking is still rather stiff and jerky, and to help with stability the arms are bent, level with the upper part of the body.

Her increasing motor abilities allow the toddler to move around on her own and investigate her living space, and so, step by step, comes a loosening of the ties with caregivers. The emerging individual will goes full steam ahead; the child wants to do everything herself. Coming to terms with a second person comes increasingly to the fore, one sign of this being the word 'No!' The defiance phase is beginning.

At this time of life the course is set that will determine how fit and skilful the child will later become. Now there is an 'up' and a 'down' and the world looks quite different. Compared to life on all fours, moving on two legs is quite different – less stable to begin with, but with a better view of things. A completely new motor challenge – but also a distinct expansion of the radius of movement, and with it an extended horizon of experience. Conscious of her own body and abilities, she strives towards higher things: she begins to climb, and so is able, for the first time all by herself, to gain a lookout onto her world. That boosts her sense of self-worth and satisfaction.

Nevertheless, at this time the pelvis that is not yet completely upright, the high extent of the lumbar lordosis, the bent knees and hip joints, and the internal rotation of the legs with compensating flat feet all show pronounced vestiges of the all-fours persisting in the toddler. So, although the child can already stand and walk, a longer period of maturation is needed before full verticality is reached.

Table 6.1 summarises the separate sensorimotor developmental stages and socialisation of the toddler. From the energetic point of view the following development can be seen.

Within the 12 developing main meridians a direction of *ki* flow has been established, beginning with the discovery of the centre at the age of about three months. Until such time as the toddler has acquired the ability to walk independently, each set of four developing meridians works closely together as a circuit within each of the families.

By 18 months at the latest, a toddler should be able to walk on her own. The ability to stand upright is the beginning of a new orientation of the collaborating meridians, the six *keiraku* described in section 3.1 – until, at around 5 to 7 years of age, this new orientation has developed to the point where the *keiraku* level can be seen as fully developed. So at the toddler stage, although it marks the beginning of the developing meridians' new orientation in the direction of the *keiraku*, the circuit of the four 'young' meridians in a family is still dominant.

6.2 Principles of treatment

The dominance of movement via the circuits during this phase of development is also the reason for doing treatment at the level of the family (and not the *keiraku*) in the case of a disorder or abnormality (i.e. the stroking technique for treating the meridians is done on the circuit of the family concerned).

In the following example of Jonah, aged 20 months, I wish to illustrate the importance of looking closely and taking any accompanying family circumstances into account, so as to identify correctly the meridians of the family where the cause of the problem lies. This example is also meant to give an idea of the skills that a Shōnishin acupuncturist needs in everyday practice. Besides knowledge of child and energetic development, a good approach to talking to the parents, and frequently painstaking detective work are also required in order to put one's finger on the key to an issue. In the example given here, treatment actually started off on the wrong tack.

Table 6.1: Sensorimotor and social development of toddlers

Age	Socialisation	Motor skills
18–24 months	Emergence of individual will is going full steam ahead: wants to do everything herself Confrontation with the 'other' comes more and more to the fore: • saying 'No!' • beginning of the defiance phase • spending more time playing alone • beginning to show sympathy, but also pretence	Standing: • standing up • good balance Walking: • walking independently, still rather stiff and jerky • arms sometimes raised • many associated movements • able to walk backwards • going up/down stairs while holding on to something Hands: • pincer grip • using cup/spoon independently
2 years	Increasingly detached from caregiver, thanks to: • increasing motor competencies • ability to move around and away freely • playing with other children • playing alone in a room when mother absent Crux in development of sense of self: • saying, 'No!' • developing self-awareness – recognising self in a mirror	Standing: • many varied transitional movements when getting up off the floor and standing • squatting to pick things up • kicking a ball in standing position Walking: • walking with ease and 'flow' • swinging arms • running confidently • few associated movements • going up/down stairs more or less confidently Hands: • can turn separate pages of a book • skilful at unwrapping sweets

Example: delayed development

Jonah, 20 months old, is the younger of two brothers. I was asked to treat him because he was not yet walking. The pregnancy and birth had been normal. His mother said he was easy to look after. Neurological disorder could be ruled out as a reason for his delayed development. Because he showed no sign of any disorder of the centre, the front family could be ruled out as the energetic cause.

Therefore I judged that a disorder in the *back* family was the reason for the deficiency in the upright dimension, this being the family with special responsibility for becoming upright. After three sessions (basic treatment, meridian treatment, back family yuan points), which Jonah very much enjoyed (and always liked to be repeated several times), there was no sign of any improvement in his motor abilities. At this point I did a further, rather more detailed observation of his movement.

It now struck me that Jonah didn't move very much at all: I would put him down on the floor and there he sat, apparently contented – I placed a rattle a little way away from him, but he gave no sign of moving. He only raised his arm to point at the rattle with a 'da-da!' and immediately his mother came and handed him the rattle. I asked her if she brought everything to him in the same way at home. She said yes, laughing as she told me that he had the whole family at his beck and call.

I asked his mother to see things for a moment through Johah's eyes. Then I put the rattle down next to him, a small distance away. This appeared to make no impression on him, and so he made no move towards it. Not until I put the rattle down in front of him did he react by pointing his finger at it and smiling to indicate that I should pick it up. When I failed to react to his pointing finger, after a while he attempted to reach the rattle. What then struck me was that he attempted to do so in the same sitting position as before, shuffling towards the rattle on his bottom.

I put him onto all fours and managed only with his mother's car key to persuade him to move forwards – and then not by crawling, but with a 'rabbit hop', where he supported himself on his arms, sliding forwards on his knees, both legs at once. It was obvious that he was avoiding (or had no experience of) shifting weight with shortening of the body on one side, and movement transitions. He always remained in whichever position he was in.

The lack of rotation in the upper body in order to reach for something, and the avoidance of the rotation that is essential for crawling, proved to me that his *lateral* family had so far failed to develop – and this despite the fact that the prerequisite for rotation, that is, discovery of one's own centre, had been met. In answer to my inquiry his mother said that as a baby Jonah had disliked lying on his front and therefore was hardly ever put down on his tummy. But as early as four months he was sitting, which he was able to do very well.

In my continuing diagnostic procedure the following two aspects were important:

1. Jonah was not sufficiently well motivated to explore himself and his potential for movement.

2. The most important movement that he needed in order to explore and master his own movement potential and ability, and the space around him, was rotation – just the one he lacked.

I explained to his mother how important it is to motivate a child to move, and treated Jonah twice for the lateral family. His mother rang to cancel the third appointment because Jonah was beginning to pull himself up by chairs and tables. When I asked, she described the way he did this first by putting one leg forward and then the other. This meant that in order to get up and pull himself up he had to lengthen (extend) one side and shorten (flex) the other. And he would get back down on the floor in the same way – first kneeling with one leg, and then the other. This is exactly the quality of the lateral family.

This example demonstrates very clearly how important it is not to rely on a single result but to look more closely, ask specific questions and examine critically.

Remember!

- For the conditions and disorders discussed here, the suggested supplementary treatments listed along with the basic treatment should be understood as suggestions only. Every single case must be given individual consideration, as the example of Jonah shows!

6.3 Conditions and disorders

Typical disorders at the toddler stage are:

- bronchitis (see also section 7.3)

- *kanmushi*

- inflammation of the middle ear (otitis media) (see also section 7.3)

- neurodermatitis (see also section 7.3)

- sleep disturbance (see also section 7.3)

- digestive problems (see section 7.3).

Bronchitis

An infection in the upper respiratory tract can spread to the mucous membranes of the lower respiratory tract. Toddlers in particular may develop severe symptoms. The cause is usually viruses, which often cause colds as well. If, as frequently happens, bacteria settle on the damaged mucous membrane after a few days, purulent bronchitis can develop.

SUPPLEMENTARY TREATMENT

- Meridian treatment of the front family

- Source points of the front family

- Vibration treatment in the region of Du 14

- Stroking treatment on the lung projection field, in particular lung areas Lu 1 and Lu 2 (Figure 6.1)

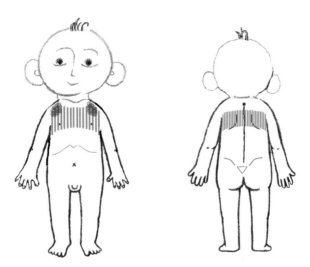

Figure 6.1

- Gentle tapping on the area of the reaction zone according to M. Tanioka (Figure 6.2)

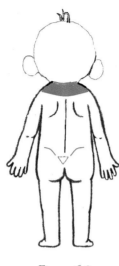

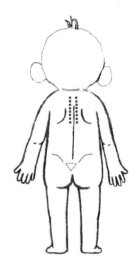

Figure 6.2   *Figure 6.3*

- Gentle tapping (from cranial to caudal) in the area of the bladder meridian from Bl 11 to Bl 18 (Figure 6.3)

Kanmushi

For crying at night, traditional advice from *Sacks of Wisdom and Oceans of Knowledge* recommends:

> Either rub a sparse application of cobra lilies into the palm of the child's hand, or write a magic sign in red on the child's navel; otherwise write the signs for 'older brother of Fire/Tiger' in red on a piece of paper and place it beside the pillow – in a wondrous way, the crying will cease.
>
> Other possibilities: smear aralia burnt to ash over the mother's breast when breastfeeding; or mix powdered motherwort into the milk and feed it to the child. This is also effective: a little earth from the middle of a path and from the kitchen stove, pounded fine and mixed with water fresh from the well, given to drink. (Rotermund 2010)

On *kanmushi*, M. Tanioka writes:

> Kanmushi is not a special name for a condition or disease; rather it is the current Japanese term for a variety of symptoms in little children aged between 3 months and 5 years.
>
> An important aspect in diagnosis of kanmushi is the child's facial expression. If the child is in good spirits, smiling, and has a typical child's face, kanmushi is scarcely visible. If the child has a wily, sharp look and the face appears small, this is a pronounced sign of kanmushi.

The faces of children with kanmushi are often pale; the circulation of blood is poor. Between the eyebrows and in the area around the bridge of the nose an angry vein can often be seen. If the condition gets worse, an angry vein can also appear at the outer corners of the eyes. The conjunctiva is blue (for example), the child has an inflamed eyelid; the outside of the nostrils and the area below the nose are red.

The main symptoms are crying at night, a squeaky voice, trying to bite other people, banging the head against objects or all manner of places, frequent crying, loss of appetite, constipation, frequent high temperature and coughing, also cramp. From the viewpoint of modern medicine one can suppose that kanmushi is some kind of neurological disorder in little children. Lack of parental affection, or life circumstances around the child, also play a large part.

The job of an acupuncture treatment is to bring forth and support the natural healing force that exists within a living body, and with Shōnishin an effect of this kind can be seen in almost all complaints. Above all, because little children are full of vital force, even a tiny stimulation can produce an astonishing effect.

With kanmushi too, there are severe and mild cases, just as there are acute and mild illnesses. Depending on the disorder, there are differences in degree, from severe to mild. Of course it is also possible to read the degree of kanmushi in the facial expression of the child. (Wernicke 2009)

Milder forms of *kanmushi* would most probably not be treated in the Western world. Dealing with a dynamic, stubborn child is certainly not easy, but it is pretty unlikely that it would be seen as a reason for doing therapy.

Here we must keep the Japanese situation in mind:

Because of light building construction and the density of housing in Japan, flats and houses are generally very permeable to noise. As *kanmushi* occurs mainly at night and the affected child is far from quiet, the noise level causes huge stress for the parents. One doesn't want to be a burden to the neighbours, after all! Being a burden to someone else – Japanese cultural practice won't allow it. Therefore *kanmushi* becomes a problem in need of treatment.

In short, *kanmushi* means a whimpering, irritable and defiant child. The fact that the parents of such children play a role here (in terms of 'parenting style') is clear to paediatricians and practitioners of traditional medicine in Japan, as elsewhere. To them *kanmushi* can be seen more as the outcome of the mother's attitude towards her baby, which is typically insecure and over-solicitous.

It was different in ancient Japan in the Tokugawa era: at that time it was supposed that evil spirits entered the child and made her unruly. Although corporal punishment of children was the exception then as now (see Chapter 1), at the time *mushifuji*, a priestly ceremony, would occasionally be performed with such a child. A powder, presumably moxa, was burnt on the child's skin to drive away the evil spirits (Herold 1993).

Nowadays, thank goodness, we have Shōnishin and practices reminiscent of exorcism are a thing of the past! Today in modern Japan *kanmushi* is seen as a disorder that requires treatment, and is also the most frequently given diagnosis. The following procedure has proved its efficacy as an adjunct to the basic treatment for *kanmushi*.

SUPPLEMENTARY TREATMENT

In the supine position:

- Repeated stroking in the area of the cranio–cervical transition (especially Bl 10, Gb 20)

- Vibration treatment on the region of He 7

- Permanent needle at Bl 15

- Tapping treatment on the area of the reaction zone according to M. Tanioka (Figure 6.4)

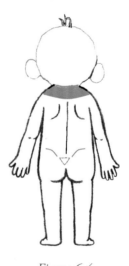

Figure 6.4

Inflammation of the middle ear (otitis media)

Traditional advice from *Sacks of Wisdom and Oceans of Knowledge* suggests:

> If there is discharge from the ear, dissolve alum over the fire, roast a little lead oxide, grind it all up finely, take a bamboo tube and blow a bit into the ear, three or five times a day. Or lightly apply the charred skin of a cricket

dispersed in sesame oil. If there is bleeding [from the ear], blow powdered dragon bones into the ear. (Rotermund 2010)

If a child is restless, cries a lot, is refusing food and constantly grabbing at the same ear, this may indicate inflammation of the middle ear. Ninety per cent of the time it is caused by viruses in the oral cavity that invade the middle ear and start an inflammation there.

FLUID BEHIND THE EARDRUM

The passage between the middle ear and the pharynx serves to ventilate the tympanic cavity. In children under seven this canal is still very short, straight and narrow. If infections, allergies or enlarged tonsils cause inflammation and swelling of the mucous membranes, the passage can become closed up and secretion cannot flow through. This can lead to painless accumulation of fluid behind the eardrum.

Often there is no obvious sign of this. There is cause for suspicion if the child is hard of hearing, either permanently or recurrently, in one or both ears, complaining of pressure in the ear, or suffering from a chronic cold. If hearing is impaired for a very long this can lead to problems with speech and language development, especially in younger children.

SUPPLEMENTARY TREATMENT

- Repeated stroking over the area of the cranio–cervical transition (especially Bl 10, Gb 20, SJ 17)

- Stroking over the whole of the area behind the sternocleidomastoid muscle

- Stroking treatment on the lung projection field and Lu 1 and Lu 2 (Figure 6.5)

- Repeated stroking over the reaction zone according to M. Tanioka – especially along the front lymph belt (Figure 6.6)

- Gentle tapping treatment over the reaction zone according to M. Tanioka – especially along the back lymph belt (Figure 6.7)

- Fluid behind the eardrum: additional tapping treatment around C7 (Figure 6.8)

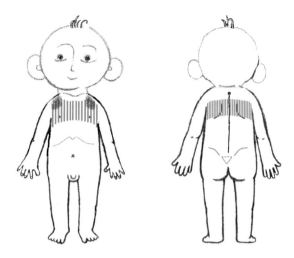

Figure 6.5

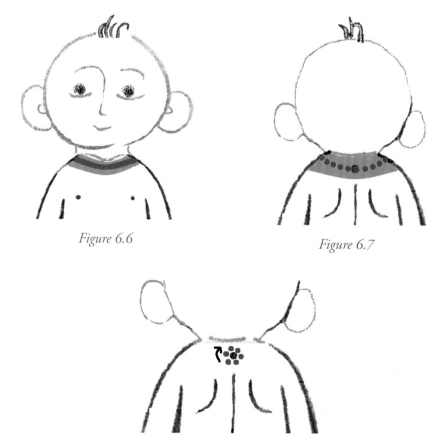

Figure 6.6

Figure 6.7

Figure 6.8

Neurodermatitis

Hardly any other illness is the subject of so much half-knowledge and misinformation as neurodermatitis. One such mistake is the belief that neurodermatitis is usually a food allergy. What is true is that a certain variety of foods can occasionally trigger a flare-up of neurodermatitis.

The incidence of neurodermatitis has increased in recent decades. Nowadays around one child in ten has the symptoms. Typical are, first, patches of dry, blotchy, mostly very itchy skin, which can become crusty with scratching, or else turn into wet, bright red or bleeding wounds. In toddlers it predominantly affects the head (cheeks, eyebrows, behind the ears), neck, shoulders and the extensor sides of the arms and legs. In older children the eczema appears on the face, throat and back of the neck, but mainly on the elbows and the backs of the knees. In adolescents the hands and feet are often also affected.

Genetically determined hypersensitivity has been shown to be the cause. Owing to limited ability to retain water, the skin is drier and thus more permeable to pathogens. This makes it more susceptible to irritation. A flare-up of neurodermatitis can be set off by food, mites, pollen, animal hair, cigarette smoke or a dry, centrally heated atmosphere. The wide range of triggers are all very different in character. What all neurodermatitis sufferers have in common, however, is that 'psychological stress' is a trigger.

Please note:

- As genetic factors play a part in neurodermatitis the predisposition to eczema is present from birth, even if it manifests only later (after weeks, months or even years), and treatment will always be on the level of the three families (i.e. treatment on the circuits from the toddler stage onwards).

- Caution: Do not treat affected skin – touch can cause or aggravate itching.

SUPPLEMENTARY TREATMENT

- Meridian treatment: front family

- Source points: front family

- Gentle tapping over the reaction zone according to M. Tanioka (Figure 6.9)

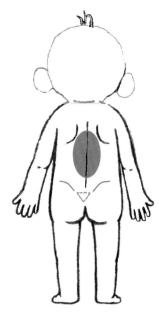

Figure 6.9

Tip

- In babies and toddlers the skin is highly sensitive. In the bath the skin swells and becomes dry, and so more vulnerable to infection by bacteria. Therefore:

    ○ Limit baths to once a week.

    ○ The bath should last for no more than 7–10 minutes.

    ○ The water temperature should be 36–37°C.

    ○ Add a few drops of olive oil to the bathwater if the skin is especially dry.

Sleep disturbance

Traditional advice from *Sacks of Wisdom and Oceans of Knowledge* suggests:

> To prevent insomnia in children, place the skull bones of a marmot [or mole] next to the pillow. (Rotermund 2010)

It is often difficult to put toddlers to bed, as they may not want to be separated from either their mother or father, and the day may have been an exciting one. Two- or three-year-olds will go more or less willingly to bed if they are tired, but then they often won't go to sleep because (for example) they are still thinking about the day's experiences, or they can see ghosts or have other fears. Difficulty falling asleep is exacerbated by excitement during the day, or if the environment is unfamiliar.

Tips

- The child should not experience tension or excitement before bedtime.

- Finish the day with a ritual – the same one every time! It may be possible to prevent sleep problems using various relaxation techniques to create the right atmosphere for going to sleep.

- Whether or not the child suffers from nightmares or night terrors, it is important for the parents to keep calm. If fear of wild animals, ghosts or similar is stopping the child from going to sleep, then the parents should take it absolutely seriously. A dream-catcher over the bed, a magic spray (e.g. water in a plant spray with a mist nozzle) magic powder (a salt sprinkler filled with salt and rice) or a magic wand (e.g. one made from of a few straws and a piece of ribbon) can work wonders.

- If the child is woken by a nightmare, soothe the child and talk to her the next day about the subject of the dream.

SUPPLEMENTARY TREATMENT

- Vibration treatment at He 7, Li 3, Pc 7

- Bl 15 (possibly permanent needle)

- Meridian stroking technique from Ren 12 to Ren 6 (Figure 6.10)

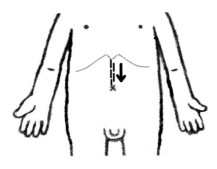

Figure 6.10

- Strong tapping in the area of the reaction zone according to M. Tanioka (Figure 6.11)

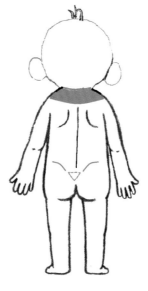

Figure 6.11

Tip

- Give a hand massage at bedtime (especially at Pc 8).

7

Treating 3–5-year-olds

The toddler stage is followed by early childhood (age 3 to 5), middle childhood (age 6 to 9) and late childhood (age 10 to 13). In many countries, early childhood is the period when the child is at nursery or kindergarten.

7.1 Sensorimotor and energetic principles

What mainly distinguishes early childhood with regard to motor development is differentiation of the motor abilities. Now, thanks to the motor confidence she has gained, the child can start to experiment: balancing along low walls, tree trunks and kerbstones, hopping on one leg, jumping with both legs together off the bottom step of the staircase, and learning to use a scooter or tricycle.

At 3 the child already has the skill to stand on one leg for at least two seconds. She can also walk on tiptoe and on her heels, and go upstairs and downstairs with alternate legs without holding on to anything. At 4 she can stand on one leg for at least five seconds, and at 5 she should also be able to do a 'jumping jack'. A 6-year-old should be able to ride a bicycle without stabilisers.

These motor skills become possible thanks to the developing power in the large buttock muscles (*gluteus maximus*) allowing full extension of the hip joints and fully erect posture of the trunk. This ensures stability and confidence in the vertical position. Complete verticality, however, is not gained until after the age of 6 years.

Socialisation develops markedly from age 3. The defiance stage wears off, and the child learns to cooperate at play. She also enjoys helping with housework or in the garden, and imitates adult activities.

At 4 the child is increasingly aware of the differences between individual family members and herself as an autonomous 'I' and starts to show interest in people outside the family group. Her willingness to share and cooperate leads to the first friendships and being part of a group.

At age 5 to 6 the child has an understanding of right and wrong, good and bad, and the emotional expressions of other children, to which she is now able to respond by helping or comforting. She can consciously tell a lie, and learns to understand that her own thoughts are different from those of other people. At 5 or 6 a sense of ownership develops, which is a reason for giving a guinea pig or a rabbit to a child of this age (but no younger).

Energetic development is characterised by the emergence of the *keiraku*. The state of motor development and social attitude are now the focus of diagnostic observation.

7.2 Principles of treatment

Problems that don't arise until this stage of development are treated via the relevant *keiraku* – so the stroking technique is done along the meridians following the course of their axis. If energetic development has failed to reach full maturity at the previous stage of development, then at this current level (the family level), treatment is done following the circuit of the affected family.

Using the example of 'motor abnormality' in 5½-year-old Robin, I want to show which aspects were significant for me in order to make a diagnosis and select the appropriate therapy.

Example: Motor abnormality

Robin was brought to me by his parents on account of his 'clumsiness'. Replying to my questions about the pregnancy and birth, his mother told me that at the start of the pregnancy she had had very severe morning sickness. The birth was ten days before term and was very quick. Otherwise, everything had been fine with Robin, including the time after birth.

My examination showed the following abnormalities:

- Standing – slight lateral inclination of the head towards the right; bilateral mobility of the cervical spine was free in all directions; the back and shoulders were rounded, and overall posture was hypotonic.

- Walking – arms hanging by the sides (defective arm swing); upper body inclined slightly forwards; standing on one leg: right, 2–3 seconds/left, 8–10 seconds (with a lot of wobbling); hopping on one leg: right, 1 metre (1–2 hops)/left, 3–4 metres; couldn't do 'jumping jack' (*either* moved only his arms *or* only his legs).

- Lying – no abnormalities.

- Sitting (with legs outstretched) – pelvis tilted backwards, with pronounced rounding of the back and shortening of the ischio-crural musculature.

The information gathered on the postural and movement patterns raised further questions, which I put to the parents after the examination. I learned that Robin had not begun to reach for objects until the age of 5 months. He had rolled from his back onto his front at 7 or 8 months, but always rolled to the same side and 'it always looked very funny', said his mother. He had never crawled, but at 9 months was already pulling himself up all over the place and at the same age he was 'walking'. When I asked whether he was actually walking on his own, I was told that he walked only while holding onto things or holding his father's or mother's hand. He could walk by himself at 17 months.

The following comments show how important the last-mentioned items of information were for planning therapy:

> It was obvious that Robin had not found his centre as a baby. That he was only reaching for things at 5 months showed me that the hand–eye coordination necessary for this motor skill had not developed at the normal age. Another clue to the missing centre was the 'funny-looking' rotation (to one side only) that he executed in rolling from his back onto his tummy. This movement pattern, if not acquired at the appropriate age, can later present in different ways, as the child needs rotation for any form of movement (e.g. crawling, standing up, walking or running, reaching, turning away); and also for integration of the right and left sides of the body.

This suggested that several basic disorders lay at the bottom of Robin's 'clumsiness': for one, a restricted capacity for rotation, and for another a disturbed system of equilibrium, as appeared in the test situation. Both abnormalities are features arising from an underdeveloped lateral family – as in Robin's presentation.

That treatment is not done on the level of the lateral family – at least, not exclusively – can be seen from the previous history. The intact front family, which allows discovery of the centre, is the precondition for full emergence of the lateral family. What it comes down to is that without the centre (hand-to-hand- and foot-to-foot contact), the centre cannot be crossed, as is necessary to execute rotation.

So to begin with I treated Robin three times, at weekly intervals, via the front family and always by the same method: basic treatment, circuit treatment of the front family and of its yuan points, and tapping treatment of the spleen zone in the *hara* region. Then I left an interval of four weeks. At the fourth appointment, seven weeks after the first one, I examined Robin again.

Both his parents and I were struck by the fact that in the meantime he had started swinging his arms when he walked. The forward inclination in his upper body posture was less than on first examination. Standing on one leg and hopping were unchanged; he was still insecure in both, performing them with a lot of compensatory movement and a distinct difference between the two sides. Similarly, he was still unable to do 'jumping jack', although his parents kept practising it with him at home.

During the next three sessions, which I did in the weekly rhythm, the lateral family was the focus of treatment. If there turned out to be no significant improvement in the course of this second stage of treatment, then it would be appropriate to go for physiotherapy or psychomotor support. A week after the third treatment, Robin proudly showed me 'jumping jack' – almost perfect. Then I tested his standing on one leg, which was as follows: right, 7–8 seconds standing (compared to 2–3 seconds previously), with only slight wobbling; left, up to 20 seconds (compared to 8–10 seconds previously), with no wobbling worth mentioning. He could hop for 3 metres on his right leg (previously 1 metre) and 5 metres on his left leg (there was not enough space to go any further).

As I could no longer see any evidence of 'clumsiness', I gave up any idea of involving physiotherapy or occupational therapy. On the family level there appeared to have been 'late maturation' of the meridians, as his movement and postural patterns were now appropriate for his age. I still needed to deal with the spatial balance of the right and left sides of his body, which is to say that there was precision work to be done on coordination. Therefore I decided on three more Shōnishin treatments with the main emphasis on the lateral *keiraku,* so that he could execute the movement patterns bilaterally.

At the follow-up examination three months after the final treatment Robin had a harmonious gait and his posture indicated self-awareness. The previous week, he had started learning aikido.

Robin's example shows how important it is to meet a child on his existing level of energetic development. This generates the assumption that the meridians can make up for delayed development. Otherwise, at best, nothing will happen or – a less favourable scenario – the child will refuse to cooperate because the demand seems too great.

If at the beginning the parents had told me that Robin had discovered his centre as appropriate for his age, and had also crawled and learned to stand by putting one foot in front of the other, then I assume that I would have begun by treating him straightaway on the level of the *keiraku.* In that case the family themes would obviously have developed in an age-appropriate way, and accordingly 'clumsiness' would only have appeared later on, that is, during the developmental stage of the *keiraku.*

Remember!

As before, in the following conditions and disorders the suggested supplementary treatments listed alongside the basic treatment should be understood purely as suggestions. As always, every case must be considered and treated on its own account.

7.3 Conditions and disorders

Problems occurring, or appearing for the first time in 3–5-year-olds in particular, are:

- asthma
- tummy ache
- bronchitis (see also section 6.3)
- enuresis (see section 8.3)
- inflammation of the middle ear (otitis media) (see also section 6.3)
- neurodermatitis (see also section 6.3)
- sleep disturbance (see also section 6.3)
- tonsillitis
- digestive problems.

Asthma

The bronchial walls are particularly sensitive in their reactions to stimuli, especially in children. Their numerous tiny muscles have a pronounced tendency to cramp, leading to frequent attacks of coughing. Constant inflammation in the bronchial tubes leads to swelling of the mucous membranes, and large quantities of thick phlegm are produced. The airways become constricted, bringing on an asthma attack.

Asthma (and neurodermatitis) is the commonest chronic illness in children – it affects over 10 per cent of all children. Onset of the disease is especially frequent between the ages of 2 and 4 years.

SUPPLEMENTARY TREATMENT

- Gentle stroking on the reaction zone according to M. Tanioka (Figure 7.1)

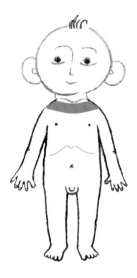

Figure 7.1

- Stroking treatment on the lung projection field, especially lung areas Lu 1 and Lu 2 (Figure 7.2)

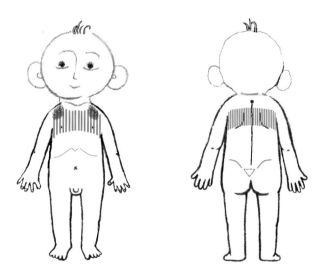

Figure 7.2

- Gentle tapping on the reaction zone according to M. Tanioka (Figure 7.3)

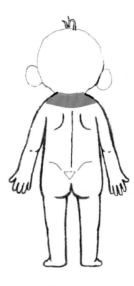

Figure 7.3

- Gentle tapping (from cranial to caudal) in the area of the Bl meridian from Bl 11 to Bl 18 (Figure 7.4)

- Vibration technique at Du 14

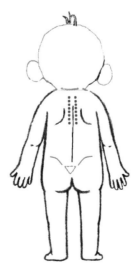

Figure 7.4

Tummy ache

In children, tummy ache occurs frequently. Whether it is really tummy ache is uncertain, as it is not always connected with the abdomen. The smaller the child, the more common it is for other parts of the body, or psychic tensions, to hurt in the region of the navel, the central point in the body. Rather, the actual cause of the tummy ache is indicated by the accompanying symptoms: bloating, cramp and diarrhoea during or after meals suggest intolerance to lactose, cows' milk or gluten; nausea and vomiting suggest involvement of the stomach; a temperature suggests inflammation as the cause.

As a rule, as long as the child is able to sit, play or jump without discomfort, there is no cause for concern. However, if tummy ache continues for more than six hours and the child's general condition is deteriorating, or if the abdomen is very hard and hurts when firmly touched, then it is essential to consult a doctor.

SUPPLEMENTARY TREATMENT

- If there is an imbalance in the child's condition:

  - treatment of the front family meridians

  - front family source points

  - stroking treatment on the stomach projection field (Figure 7.5)

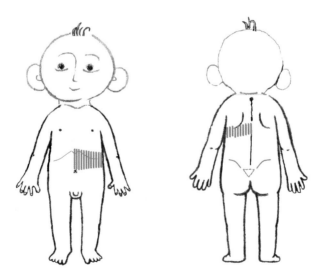

Figure 7.5

- If there are digestive problems:

  - treatment of the back family meridians

  - back family source points

  - stroking treatment on the small intestine projection field (Figure 7.6)

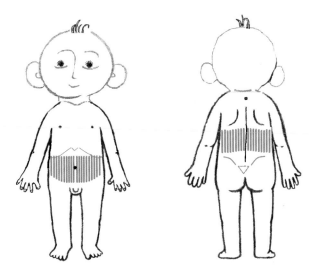

Figure 7.6

- If there is rage or anger:

  - treatment of the lateral family meridians

  - lateral family source points

Bronchitis

As a rule, acute bronchitis swiftly runs its course within a week or two, with no further problems. A longer-lasting, persistent cough indicates hypersensitive airways, which can lead to chronic inflammation of the respiratory tract. If, in addition to inflammation, there is narrowing of the bronchi, we are dealing with obstructive (spastic) bronchitis. This is characterised by impaired breathing, with wheezing on inhalation.

- See section 6.3

Inflammation of the middle ear (otitis media)

Inflammation of the middle ear usually begins with a cold. As the passage between the ear and the nose and throat is still very narrow in children, it is quickly blocked by swelling if there is inflammation, so that the middle ear secretions cannot flow away. This creates pressure against the eardrum from the inside, and leads to severe earache with stabbing or throbbing pain. The combination of cough, cold and earache is typical. In smaller children the trouble can also be unspecific, with the earache manifesting as tummy ache.

If the pressure on the eardrum gets too intense, it can rupture. This lets the fluid out, so the pain rapidly abates.

SUPPLEMENTARY TREATMENT

- See section 6.3

Neurodermatitis

In contrast to the toddler, the skin eruption in the kindergarten child is less wet, scalier and drier and often marked by scratching.

SUPPLEMENTARY TREATMENT

- See section 6.3

Sleep disturbance

Children as young as 2 can suffer from nightmares: from the age of 3 onwards these can occur more frequently and wake the child up in fright.

One particular form of night-time anxiety is attacks of 'night terrors' (*pavor nocturnus*), which can occur after the age of 2. These terror attacks occur during phases of deep sleep. The child utters bloodcurdling screams, thrashes around, kicks and appears very frightened, looking around wildly with open eyes – but without waking up.

Whether or not the child suffers from nightmares or night terrors, it is important for the parents to keep calm. If fear of wild animals, ghosts or similar is stopping the child from falling asleep, then the parents should take it absolutely seriously.

SUPPLEMENTARY TREATMENT

- See section 6.3

Tips

- A dream-catcher over the bed, a magic spray (e.g. water in a plant spray with a mist nozzle), magic powder (a salt sprinkler filled with salt and rice) or a magic wand (e.g. one made from a few straws and a piece of ribbon) can work wonders.

- With night terrors the child is not awake, but can be assisted by placing any pointed objects out of reach to prevent the child injuring themselves while thrashing around.

Tonsillitis

Pharyngeal inflammations are among the commonest illnesses for 3–5-year-olds. The causes are almost exclusively viral or bacterial. Tonsillitis is typically characterised by sore throat and painful swallowing with a sense of constriction in the throat. There is reddening of the oral cavity and the tonsils are swollen and may be covered in pustules.

SUPPLEMENTARY TREATMENT

- Meridian treatment of the front family

- Front family source points

- Vibration treatment at Gb 34

- Tapping treatment around C7 (Figure 7.7)

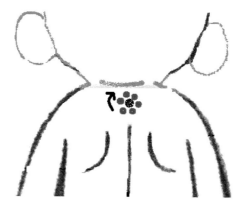

Figure 7.7

- Repeated stroking in the area of the cranio-cervical transition (especially Bl 10, Gb 20, SJ 17)

- Gentle tapping treatment on the reaction zone according to M. Tanioka, especially along the back lymph belt (Figure 7.8)

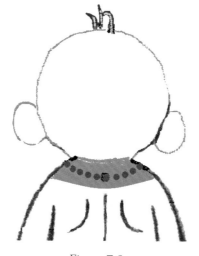

Figure 7.8

Tip

- Apply a potato poultice on the neck to ease inflammation.

Digestive problems

Diarrhoea

Diarrhoea is mostly a natural reaction of the digestive system, the body's way of clearing itself of pathogens. In chronic forms there is often a functional disorder of the intestines or damage to the intestinal flora (e.g. following treatment with antibiotics).

If diarrhoea is linked with cramp-like pains, there may be intolerance of milk sugar (lactose) or fruit sugar (fructose). Intolerance of cows' milk should also be considered as a possible cause of diarrhoea.

If there is vomiting in addition to diarrhoea there is the risk of dehydration, which is particularly dangerous for babies and toddlers. Therefore the most important thing is to replace fluid and minerals.

Supplementary treatment

- Meridian treatment of the front family

- Front family source points

Or use:

- Back family meridian treatment and source points (if there is agitation, fear, nervous strain)

- Vibration treatment (possibly also permanent needle) in the area of St 25, on both sides

In either case, continue with:

- gentle tapping treatment around the navel – anticlockwise (Figure 7.9)

- tapping treatment above the crest of the pelvis – from the centre outwards, as in the basic treatment (Figure 7.10)

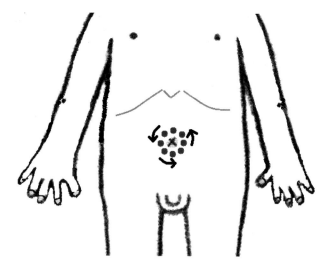

Figure 7.9

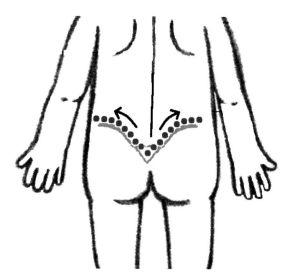

Figure 7.10

- gentle tapping on the bladder meridian, from Bl 20 to Bl 25 (Figure 7.11)

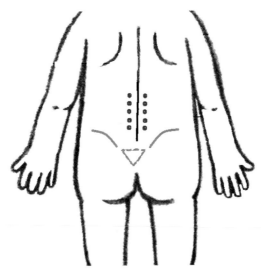

Figure 7.11

- gentle tapping in the area of the reaction zone according to M. Tanioka (Figure 7.12)

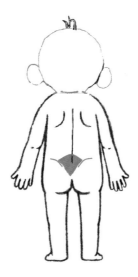

Figure 7.12

- stroking treatment on the small intestine projection field (Figure 7.13)

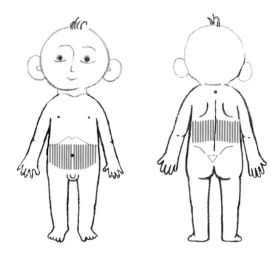

Figure 7.13

CONSTIPATION

Constipation often occurs at the toilet-training stage. For fear of missing the right moment to go to the toilet, and then soiling her pants, the child holds back stools. If constipation goes on for long, stools thicken to the point where passing them can be very painful. Then there is fear of pain as well, and so the child waits as long as possible before next going to the toilet – the beginning of a vicious circle.

A further cause of constipation lies in the fact that children, like many adults, have sensitive reactions to external influences such as, for example, a new daily routine, unfamiliar surroundings (holiday) or dirty toilets.

SUPPLEMENTARY TREATMENT

- Meridian treatment of the back family (if fear of pain is the key factor)

- Vibration treatment of back family source points (fear of pain)

- Stroking treatment on the kidney/bladder projection field (Figure 7.14)

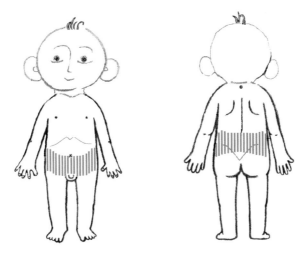

Figure 7.14

Or use:

- Meridian treatment of the front family (if constipation is provoked by external influences)

- Vibration treatment of front family source points (if provoked by external influences)

- Vibration treatment at St 25 on both sides

- Stroking treatment on the large intestine projection field (Figure 7.15)

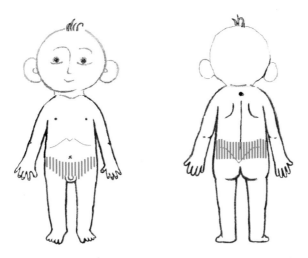

Figure 7.15

In either case, continue with:

- Gentle tapping treatment around the navel (Figure 7.16)

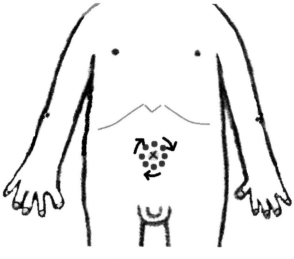

Figure 7.16

- Tapping treatment above the crest of the pelvis (Figure 7.17)

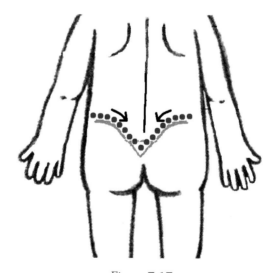

Figure 7.17

- Gentle tapping on the bladder meridian from Bl 20 to Bl 25 (Figure 7.18)

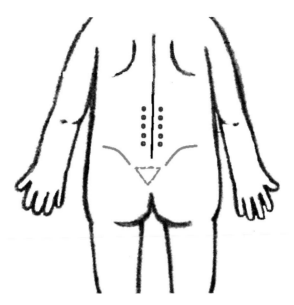

Figure 7.18

- Gentle tapping in the area of the reaction zone according to M. Tanioka (Figure 7.19)

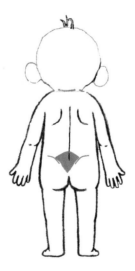

Figure 7.19

8

Treating 6–13-year-olds

The child has left early childhood behind and is now entering middle childhood (age 6 to 9 years), which is then followed by late childhood (age 10 to 13 years).

8.1 Sensorimotor and energetic principles

Motor development has now reached a stage where the child is beginning to work harder at refining and specialising motor skills. She is discovering ambition in sport, not just play any more – what matters increasingly are her expectations of her own abilities.

So at the sports club, for example, she devotes herself to the sport she likes the most. It may be a competitive team sport; or one in which she asserts herself more as the 'sole competitor'; or maybe sporting activities that demand more in terms of stamina or dexterity. Agility, physical mobility, strength, speed or tests of physical endurance are the physical challenges that the child is now specifically seeking. At the same time there is the process of identifying with their own gender, with increasingly gender-specific behaviour. Teachers and classmates become new 'significant others'.

On the emotional level there is a process of 'refinement'. Sudden, unfiltered expressions of emotion are becoming better adapted to given situations and more finely nuanced. This means that the child is able to adjust her 'inner world' adequately for the 'outside world' and to perceive the outside world in a more differentiated way – in other words: there is improvement in the child's social competence.

This is also happening on the energetic plane: up to now, the *keiraku* have been in the forefront. The up–down connections of the yin–yang meridians provided the energetic foundation for the new motor experience of being upright. By the end of this developmental stage all the basic movement patterns are running 'automatically'. The child is now able to stand on one leg and hop, climb a tree, walk backwards, balance and ride a bicycle – to give just a few examples.

In order to adapt the inner world to the outside world on the meridian level, the 'inner' yin meridians are becoming increasingly orientated towards the 'outer' yang meridians, and vice versa. So emotional expression is conveyed to the outside world via the yin meridians, and the surrounding world's reaction to this expression is passed to the inside via the yang meridians. This experience helps shape the child's future behaviour. An example:

The child expresses her anger with another child via the liver meridian – stupidly, as the other child is taller by a head – and so the gallbladder meridian finds out what it is like to get a black eye, and tells the liver meridian, 'Next time, think a bit more about when and how you get angry!'

Now the five phases are in their element. Nevertheless, the energetic links between 'family' and *keiraku* still exist:

- The three families are, and remain, the resources on which the child (and later the adult) can draw, and which give her strength. So from front family experience the child learns that 'I am worthy of attention', and also the power and strength to give a talk in front of the whole class. Or – as an example relating to the back family – from the experience that 'it's OK for me to take a break' the child acquires a sense of when she needs a rest, and gives herself permission to do so.

- By age 6 all six *keiraku* should be interacting to make economical sequences of movement available for daily living. So the child is able to lean down from her chair to get a book out of her bag without falling off her chair and without creating a noise. Or – to give another example – the child should be able to write for the duration of a full lesson, sitting up, and without fidgeting.

So, depending on a given situation, the schoolchild can draw on the appropriate energetic link (family, *keiraku*, phase). But she cannot do so if the energetic link failed to reach maturity at the appropriate developmental stage (family – up to the time of being able to walk independently; *keiraku* – after learning to walk up to ages 5–6; phase – from age 6 onward).

8.2 Principles of treatment

If a problem arises – and the same applies to adults – we need to see which stage of energetic development the presenting issue belongs to. Depending on the stage of energetic development at which the problem first appeared, the child or adult is treated on the corresponding level. So in meridian treatment, stroking technique is done either on the pathway of the circuit of the appropriate family, or on the pathway of the axes of the appropriate *keiraku*, or on the pathway of the internal/external connection of the appropriate phase.

I would like to illustrate this with the following example. Over the past two decades the topic of ADHD has received a great deal of publicity. That is one reason why I have chosen this subject, and not least because the diagnosis of ADHD is now being used in a way that may be seen as inflationary. The case described here shows how a child can all too soon be labelled with this diagnosis. When there is a diagnosis of ADHD, the closest observation on the part of the practitioner is absolutely essential in order to steer Shōnishin treatment in the right direction.

Example: 'ADHD'

Tanya was 7 when her mother brought her to see me for the first time. She was in the second year at school. Her mother told me:

The birth had been two weeks pre-term and entirely unproblematic – although immediately after birth Tanya had to stay in hospital (with her mother) for a week because of a neonatal infection. Up until the age of 6 weeks, Tanya had been easy to look after.

Then something happened: While her father was carrying her in his arm, she suddenly woke up with a start, fell out of her father's arm at the top of the staircase, and tumbled down 13 stairs. She was taken to hospital with a fractured skull.

Following that there was a change in her behaviour. After leaving hospital, she cried constantly; she could be soothed only by being carried. In contrast to the time before the accident, she had huge problems going to sleep. Dropping off to sleep could take as long as two hours. When she finally got as far as falling asleep, if she was laid down in her cot she would instantly wake up again. She would only go to sleep properly if her mother lay down next to her, and then she would briefly wake up at intervals of one to three hours in order (her mother said) either to be breastfed or to check that everything was all right.

Her motor development was entirely normal and she was able to walk on her own at 12 months, having crawled for quite a long time. She had been able to climb very early, riding a bicycle without stabilisers by the age of 3, and swimming without buoyancy aids at 4.

The actual reason why her mother had come to consult me was her teacher's diagnosis of ADHD, which had been mentioned for the first time at kindergarten. At the time (Tanya was just 5) the ADHD diagnosis had not been confirmed by a paediatrician. But now that the teacher was assuming the diagnosis yet again, she (the mother) felt very unsure. Tanya did, in fact, seem very abnormal. As far as the sleeping problems were concerned, nothing had really changed since the accident.

So she still couldn't sleep on her own. Yes, she would go to sleep in her own bed, but there would be a lot of fuss beforehand: getting up to go to the toilet as often as five times; in between, one foot had to be massaged because it was hurting, or her back needed scratching because it was itching, she had to have a sip of water, or have her tummy stroked because she had tummy ache; then it would be too light or too dark in her room, the duvet too warm or the room too cold, etc., etc., and in the end, at some point, every night she would get into bed with her mother.

Maybe, her mother thought, this was because her father was only at home at weekends, as he worked 350 kilometres away from home. She also told me that at school (just as previously at kindergarten) Tanya would not follow any rules. At home she was also 'utterly stubborn' and would insist on having her own way, which led to big power struggles. She was the one who determined what was to be done, and when.

Another abnormality was that everything had to be 'just so'; nothing was allowed to be different. For example, two weeks previously her brother, who was five years older than her, had borrowed her chair just long enough to get something down from a cupboard. When he put the chair back next to Tanya's table, she had a tantrum that went on for hours because the chair hadn't been put back the way it was supposed to be. Her mother also experienced Tanya's 'attacks' almost every day – for example, if she had dusted Tanya's table, and biros and crayons were not lying in exactly the same place as before.

Her mother also said that Tanya kept asking whether she still loved her. Her mother had the feeling that Tanya kept overstepping boundaries in order to gain reassurance that she was still loved, even if she had 'driven me to a frazzle'.

I examined Tanya, during which she was very cooperative – even if she did have to hold her mother's hand almost the whole time. Movement and postural patterns, coordination and balance (when she did actually let go of her mother!) were all very well developed. I was able to rule out blockage of the cervical spine (e.g. as a result of the accident). She listened well and I didn't have to repeat any requests or instructions, and there were no signs of hyperactive behaviour.

Diagnosis

Her compulsive need to be close to her mother, difficulty letting go in order (for example) to go to sleep, and constant need to be reassured that she was loved – these were all back family issues. She had lost her parents' support at seven weeks – a truly traumatic experience.

TREATMENT

I carried out six Shōnishin treatments at weekly intervals. As the symptoms were obviously caused by the accident when Tanya was 7 weeks old, there had been a disturbance of the developing back family. Therefore, in addition to the basic treatment, I treated the back family circuit, and its yuan points.

RESULTS

At the second treatment Tanya's mother told me that after the first treatment Tanya had gone to bed that evening without a fuss, and had remained in her own bed until the morning. Apart from that, nothing had changed.

Over the course of the six treatments, Tanya's mother said, there had been 'not a single relapse'. It was striking, however, that whenever Tanya's father came home at the weekend, Tanya would demand reassurance more often that her father or mother loved her. During the week, when she was alone with her mother, the subject no longer arose.

At school Tanya's class teacher had noticed that her participation in lessons increased significantly. She was also (the teacher told her mother) a lot calmer.

In the normal way, I made another appointment with Tanya and her mother for a chat six weeks later. Her mother said: 'Tanya's better, I'm better, we're all feeling better and Tanya has no problems at school – we're happy!'

Remember!

As in previous chapters, in the following conditions and abnormalities the suggested supplementary treatments listed alongside the basic treatment should be understood purely as suggestions. As always, every case must be considered and treated on its own account.

8.3 Conditions and disorders

Typical abnormalities, disorders and illnesses at this stage of development are:

- asthma (see also section 7.3)

- bronchitis (see sections 6.3 and 7.3)

- enuresis (bedwetting)

- neurodermatitis (see sections 6.3 and 7.3)

- sleep disturbance (see also sections 6.3 and 7.3).

Asthma

In children of 6–13 years asthma is caused predominantly by allergies, but sometimes allergies are absent – the main triggers are infections of the respiratory tract, physical exertion or psychological stress.

SUPPLEMENTARY TREATMENT

- See section 7.3

Enuresis (bedwetting)

> For bedwetting, char the entrails of a chicken and take them with hot water: the effect is wonderful. (Rotermund 2010)

> Toilet training of children began at the age of about one-and-a-half years. Children were told that the toilet divinity would be watching them and that therefore they had to do it right. If the children had understood the lesson, they were praised. (Herold 1993)

Statistically, one in five 5-year-olds and one in ten 7-year-olds regularly or occasionally wet the bed. The term 'enuresis' is used if, after their fifth birthday, a child is not dry throughout the day and/or at night. Either the child has never been dry (primary enuresis) or after staying dry for at least six months, she has started bedwetting again (secondary enuresis). Whether enuresis is primary or secondary, it is always important to rule out organic causes.

CAUSES (THE WESTERN VIEW)

The Western view assumes the following causes:

- functional/psychological (children with enuresis have significantly more frequent fear responses)

- delayed maturity of the central nervous system (reduced secretion of vasopressin at night)

- genetic predisposition (in many families there appears to be autosomal dominant inheritance)

- (rare) organic/anatomical disorder: anatomical anomalies such as occluded ureter, spinal cord injury).

CAUSES (THE EASTERN VIEW)

In Eastern medicine two different types of energetic disorder are generally suspected to be the causes of enuresis: on the one hand deficiency of kidney yang (a disorder in the back family), which corresponds to primary enuresis; and on the other hand deficiency of spleen *ki* or possibly lung *ki* (a disorder in the front family), which corresponds to secondary enuresis.

THE BROADER DIAGNOSTIC CONTEXT

On initial examination a test is done for a persisting Galant reflex. This reflex is active chiefly during birth: in response to the stroking effect on the area of the bladder meridian at the thoraco-lumbar level it sets off a snake-like movement in the child to support or even enable the baby's passage along the birth canal (see also section 5.4).

Up to the sixth month of life, stroking an infant on both sides of the bladder meridian in the thoraco-lumbar section of its pathway will set off this Galant reflex. As a result, the child will usually immediately begin to urinate. After the sixth month at the latest, this reflex should die away, which is why it is counted as one of the early childhood reflexes. If it persists, however, the reflex can be set off in older children – during sleep, for example – which can lead to momentary loss of bladder control and bedwetting.

So, on the meridian level, the developing bladder meridian, which belongs to the back family, is responsible for the Galant reflex, its motor response and vegetative functioning; and the basic patterns of the back family, which include building up muscle tone and stability, are aspects of the Galant reflex. Not only does it have a role to play in the birth process, it is also responsible for the connection between the thorax and the pelvis, and the erect position of the spine.

If this reflex persists it can lead to weakening in the thoraco-pelvic region. This explains why persisting traces of the Galant reflex can lead, among other things, to instability of the spine, since these conditions are not the best for developing stable control of the trunk. In the same way, it can lead to functional weakness in the urogenital tract, with resultant bedwetting that may continue later than the toddler stage.

SUPPLEMENTARY TREATMENT
Meridian treatment of the back family

- Back family source points

- Vibration treatment on Du 3, Bl 28

- Vigorous tapping treatment above the pubic bone (Figure 8.1)

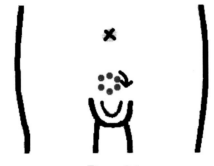

Figure 8.1

- Vigorous tapping treatment above the crest of the pelvis (Figure 8.2)

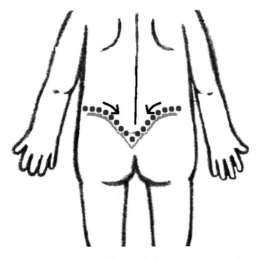

Figure 8.2

- Gentle tapping on the bladder meridian from Bl 20 to Bl 25 (Figure 8.3)

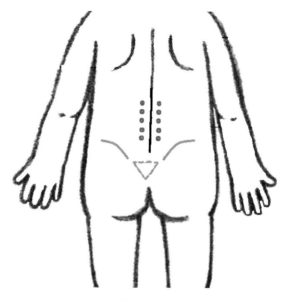

Figure 8.3

- Vigorous tapping in the area of the reaction zone according to M. Tanioka (Figure 8.4)

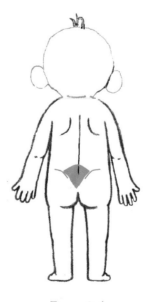

Figure 8.4

- Stroking treatment on the 'kidney–bladder' projection field (Figure 8.5)

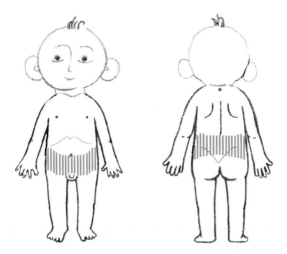

Figure 8.5

- Moxa treatment on Bl 23 (Figure 8.6)

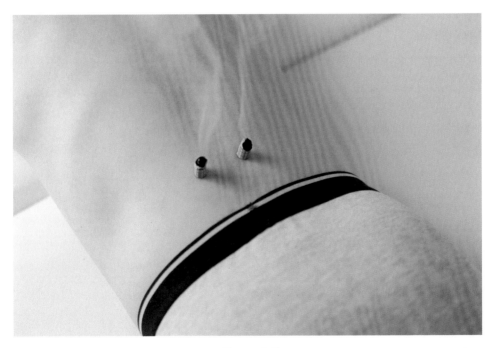

Figure 8.6

Treatment at home

- *A task for the child*: As soon as the child feels the urge to pass water, instead of going to the toilet she should go straight to her bedroom, lie down on the bed and pretend to be asleep. It is important that this is the same bed as she sleeps in at night! Draw the child's attention to the fact that this is the way her bladder feels at night when it is trying to wake her up. Then the child should wait, resisting the urge to urinate, first for one minute, the next day for one-and-a-half minutes, the day after that for two minutes, and so on, up to five minutes, before going to the toilet.

  It may be that after lying down the child no longer feels the need to urinate. This is the learning objective of pretending to be asleep, such that the effect is then unconsciously called upon during actual sleep.

  Of course, this procedure should only be done after school, at weekends and during the holidays.

- *A task for mother and/or father*: In order to extinguish the persisting Galant reflex, every night at bedtime the mother or father should roll a massage ball over the child's sacral region and along the paravertebral area of the thoraco-lumbar region, using strong but not painful pressure (Figures 8.7 and 8.8).

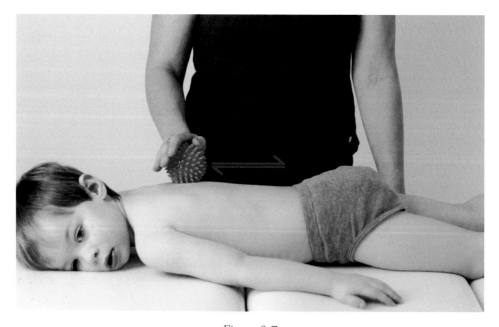

Figure 8.7

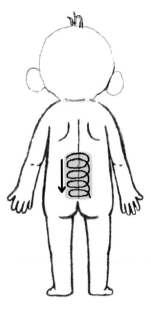

Figure 8.8

Tips

- After early evening the child should not drink large amounts of liquid.

- At bedtime make sure that the child takes enough time to pass water, so that the bladder is fully emptied.

- The subject of bedwetting should not be raised too often at home, especially when the affected child is present. This puts pressure on the child, which is counterproductive for the purpose of becoming dry.

Sleep disturbance

Nightmares become more frequent in primary-school children as the demands of school intensify. In addition, afternoon activities can gain the upper hand to such an extent that a child's engagement calendar looks like that of a manager – stressful enough, then, to have a negative impact on sleep.

In older schoolchildren the reasons for sleep disturbance are similar to those adults have in their work and personal lives – school-related troubles, difficulties with friendships and personal relationships, lack of exercise, eating too much or too late. This is exacerbated by puberty, a time when many young people feel insecure and have low self-esteem.

If sleep disturbance begins only at the stage of starting to walk, or later, and has not previously been a problem, then the treatment given is independent of the trigger that has caused it. If fear or ideation is the main factor, this indicates a disorder in the back family. This would be a case for meridian treatment of the back family in the *keiraku* pathways (supplementary to the basic treatment), and also vibration treatment of the back family source points. Feeling uprooted because of moving house, or 'upstaged' by a sibling, for example, can throw the child off centre: this is a front family theme.

At the first occurrence of sleep disturbance in a child of school age, meridian treatment is done on the level of the five phases, regardless of what is thought to be the cause of the sleep disturbance.

SUPPLEMENTARY TREATMENT

- See section 6.3

9

Treating Adults

When treating adults, as a rule needle acupuncture is preferable to Shōnishin. There are four exceptions to this, where Shōnishin is a genuine alternative option for treatment:

- if there is needle phobia
- in sensitive patients
- in patients on anticoagulant medication
- in older people.

Up to now, these patients have not been allowed to have acupuncture. The only alternatives for them have been laser acupuncture and acupressure.

A further opportunity for using Shōnishin with adults is to include it in the context of acupuncture or Shiatsu treatment. Here there are two possible options.

First, Shōnishin can be used right at the beginning of a treatment, before starting acupuncture or Shiatsu. This is particularly helpful if the patient is stressed, or comes for acupuncture or Shiatsu treatment in a state of high inner tension. The Shōnishin basic treatment 'winds down' the sympathetic nervous system very quickly, so that there is no need to wait very long before stating the actual acupuncture or Shiatsu treatment.

Second, Shōnishin can be interpolated during the last stage or at the end of a session, especially if there is tension in the neck or shoulder areas. This can be worked on directly with tapping technique. Don't forget that tapping technique feels very pleasant and is therefore particularly suitable at the end of a treatment.

9.1 Principles of treatment

As with 6–13-year-olds, with adults it is also necessary to see which stage of energetic development the presenting symptomology relates to. Here too it is important to find out when the disorder first appeared in the context of energetic development; treatment is then done at the appropriate level.

In carrying out meridian treatment, then, we can consider:

- stroking technique on the pathway of the circuit of the appropriate family, or

- stroking technique on the pathway of the internal/external connection of the appropriate phase.

Remember!

As in the treatment of children, in the following conditions and abnormalities the suggested supplementary treatments listed alongside the basic treatment should be understood purely as suggestions. As always, every case must be considered and treated on its own account.

9.2 Conditions and disorders

Shōnishin treatment has proved valuable for adults with the following abnormalities, disorders and illnesses:

- facial palsy

- urinary incontinence

- scarring.

Facial palsy

The key feature of facial palsy is paralysis on one side of the face; different causes come into consideration. A distinction is made between the peripheral and central types of paralysis. The peripheral form extends to the entire mimic musculature of one side of the face; here, incomplete closure of the eyelids is typical ('Bell's palsy'). The cause is known only in around 25 per cent of cases (e.g. Lyme disease (borreliosis), herpes zoster or tumour).

In the central form, the muscles of the forehead are not affected. Here the possible causes are mainly stroke, cerebral haemorrhage or brain tumour, and therefore this form of facial paralysis is accompanied by additional paralysis in the arm or hand.

Facial palsy is the only illness for which Shōnishin treatment is done on the face. Stroking treatment is done first on the unaffected side of the face, and then on the affected side.

Supplementary treatment

- Gentle, rapid tapping on the neck and lymph belt (see section 4.2)

- Stroking technique on the affected side of the face

- Vibration treatment on (points selected from) LI 4, SJ 5, Li 3, Gb 2–4, Gb 14, SJ 17, SJ 21–23, St 2, St 3, St 5–7, Ren 24

Urinary incontinence

Urinary incontinence is the inability to determine the exact time of passing water. The bladder is emptied involuntarily. The cause can be functional disorder of the urethral sphincter ('stress incontinence'), as frequently happens following childbirth or in old age. Here urine is passed involuntarily under physical stress, such as when carrying a heavy load, running, going upstairs or coughing or sneezing.

Another cause of urinary incontinence is cystitis. One has the feeling of needing to go to the toilet but, despite the urge to urinate, can pass only small quantities of urine. In the most pronounced form of the condition, urine can be passed involuntarily. Urinary incontinence can also occur in certain diseases – for example, Parkinson's disease, multiple sclerosis, enlarged prostate or spinal cord injury.

Urinary incontinence is a disorder that is expected in younger children but not after the age of 6 years. Seen from the perspective of energetic diagnosis, lack of bladder control would be similar to that of a child under 6, regardless of the cause in the adult. In this respect the adult has reverted to the *keiraku* level.

Supplementary treatment

- Meridian treatment: back family

- Back family source points

- Vibration treatment: Du 3, Bl 28

- Vigorous tapping treatment above the pubic bone

- Vigorous tapping treatment above the crest of the pelvis (as in the basic treatment, from the centre outwards)

- Gentle tapping on the bladder meridian from Bl 20 to Bl 25

- Gentle tapping in the area of the reaction zone according to M. Tanioka

- Moxa treatment at Bl 23

Scarring

Shōnishin's efficacy as treatment for scarring was discovered by chance:

> During my training course for midwives – in which Shōnishin training is tailored for midwifery – one of the participants asked me whether Shōnishin was also effective for relieving pain in the lower part of the body following childbirth. I had no idea and said so. She said that she was referring to herself, that she was suffering severely, and perhaps I might like to try it out on her.

> I agreed, whereupon the midwife showed me her abdomen, which was heavily scarred as a result of an emergency section 15 months earlier. I did a kinesiology test on the scars in order to gather information as to whether the scars represented an interference zone and so might be responsible for the pain. The kinesiology test was absolutely positive – evidently the scars had to be taken into account as contributing to the chronic pain, and consequently to be considered as an interference zone. After treating them with Shōnishin, I repeated the test. It was negative – but the pain in the woman's lower body continued as badly as ever.

> The following morning, shortly before the course started, the midwife came up to me. She was finding it difficult not to cry – since last night, for the first time in 15 months, she had had no pain. After the end of the course that evening I had to treat nearly all the midwives; there was scarcely one who didn't have some kind of a scar. And kinesiology testing showed that almost all the scars responded to Shōnishin.

Scars can have the characteristics of an interference zone (i.e. they can provoke disorders somewhere inside or on the body). What are we to make of this? According to Huneke, the founder of neural therapy, an interference zone disrupts the self-regulating ability of organs or muscle function chains.

Damage caused by chemical, thermal, mechanical, toxic or infectious agents brings about a disorder in the membrane potential at the cellular level. The result is a permanent false stimulus that is forwarded via sympathetic afferent nerves. These constant 'disordered' impulses upset the vegetative nervous system to such an extent that, under the influence of sympathetic efferent nerves, symptoms or disorders can arise in organs that are sometimes located far away from the actual interference zone.

With Shōnishin treatment, presumably the vegetative reaction brings about normalisation of the disrupted cell membrane potential, and hence restores harmony in the disordered vegetative nervous system. Kinesiology testing can show, for example, whether or not a scar represents an interference zone, and whether or not an interference zone has been successfully treated. Initially positive kinesiology test results, with negative results following treatment, and the relief or disappearance of symptoms that were presumably caused by the scarring/interference field, indicate successful treatment of scarring.

COMMON INTERFERENCE FIELDS

- Scars caused by:
  - Caesarean section
  - appendectomy
  - thyroidectomy
  - episiotomy
  - injuries
  - tonsillectomy
  - cosmetic surgery
  - back surgery
- tonsils (malfunctioning) or residual tissue of weak tonsils (following incomplete tonsillectomy)
- dental root treatment
- (dental) amalgam.

PROCEDURE

Since doing a series of scar treatments, the following procedure has been proven in recent years. On the head and face, and for superficial scars where there is no deep tissue (e.g. connective tissue or muscle tissue) under the scar:

- stroking treatment on the scarred area until there is a reaction (i.e. reduction of tone in the tissue directly surrounding the scar).

Scars in soft tissue:

- stroking treatment (see above), and then

- tapping treatment.

With tapping treatment the tapping should be rapid and vigorous. This is done first directly on the scar, tapping several times up and down along the scar until there is reddening (Figure 9.1). Then the tapping changes to a clockwise spiral movement, from the scar outwards (Figure 9.2).

Evidently, scars can be treated successfully with Shōnishin, in so far as they represent an interference zone and appear to be the cause of certain symptoms. Positive feedback from patients confirms this.

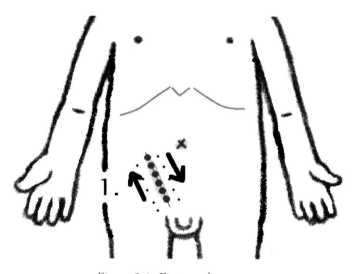

Figure 9.1: First on the scar…

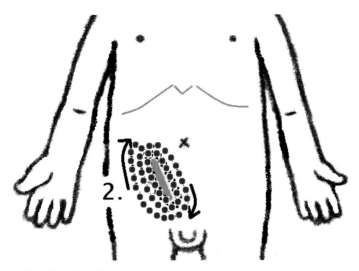

Figure 9.2: …then spiralling around the scar

10

Treating Older People with Impaired Mobility

In the next few decades we are going to see a dramatic rise in the proportion of ageing and old people, while the number of younger people is decreasing. Ageing, naturally, is linked with more or less rapid processes of deterioration. Joints wear out, muscle mass and muscle tone diminish, balance becomes increasingly shaky and mental capacity lower. These processes don't necessarily amount to illness, but all the same, the likelihood of becoming ill is higher than it is for younger adults.

For the Shōnishin acupuncturist, this opens up a large field. Experience shows that especially older people respond to Shōnishin treatment with sensitivity and gratitude. This could be because very old people have a lot in common with small children.

With advancing age their motor abilities become ever more limited, eating becomes more messy and in the end they need to be fed, bladder and bowel control is mostly inadequate, and owing to loss of short-term memory many increasingly live in the past (especially in their childhood), emotional expression becomes unstable and the skin grows thinner.

So, why not Shōnishin?

10.1 Principles of treatment

When treating old people, a few issues need to be borne in mind. These relate to the skin, communication and the way treatment is done.

THE SKIN

- Old people's skin is often like parchment, which is to say that it is thin and easily damaged. For the stroking technique the consequence is that old people should not be treated in the same way as adults, but much more gently, like children of 2 and under.

- Another skin characteristic that must be taken into account is that the older a person is, the more wrinkled their skin will be. For effective stroking treatment it is helpful to stretch the skin slightly with your non-treating hand (Figure 10.1).

COMMUNICATION

- It is important to prepare a brief, clear explanation of what you are doing, so that this generation can understand and accept treatment without anxiety. As with children, it is very important that this is framed in positive terms.

- Touch – especially with old people – is not something that should be taken for granted. Therefore, it goes without saying that what matters here is a respectful manner on the part of the Shōnishin acupuncturist. He should first request permission to touch: 'May I touch you?' This applies also – indeed, applies above all – when treating people who you think might not understand you, for example owing to advanced dementia or coma.

- Say a few words to introduce each successive step in the treatment.

- In communicating, take care to speak slowly, clearly and without running words together. Sentences should be short and simple in construction. This gives old people time to process what has been said.

DOING THE TREATMENT

- Many very old people have a strong sense of shame – so don't expect them to undress for a Shōnishin treatment. Expose only those parts of the body that are to be treated (Figure 10.2).

- Very many old people suffer from stimulus deprivation and may be hypersensitive in the way they react to stimuli. Especially those with restricted mobility perceive stimuli much more intensely than people who are inundated day in, day out, with stimuli on different levels.

Frequently they develop dysaesthesia and experience strange sensations very acutely. Therefore, in general, they also have lower pain tolerance. Because of these sensitivities, stroking treatment or vibration treatment on acupuncture points has to be done with great caution. This also applies to the rate of stroking, which is lower than it would be for younger adults.

• Bedridden patients are a special case. In their experience, everything that happens under the sheets is frequently linked with negative feelings (e.g. cleaning after soiling, inserting catheters, etc.). It's vital to take negative experiences such as these into consideration! It is therefore helpful if Shōnishin is done only on the arms and lower legs – until trust has been established. When treating the legs, only the lower part of the bed covering is pulled back. This spares the person receiving treatment the feeling that he is being laid bare.

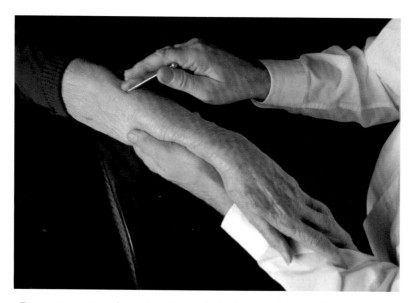

Figure 10.1: Stretching the skin with the left hand for stroking treatment

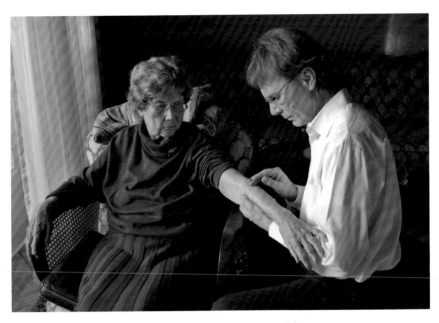

Figure 10.2: Treating a 97-year-old patient

10.2 Shōnishin for people who are seriously ill

Old people who are confined to bed have a very restricted life, and are vulnerable and helplessly at the mercy of the outside world that they depend and rely on. They need good physical care, turning to avoid pressure sores, and human contact. While physical care and turning are carried out as part of a minimum programme of care, for the most part human contact is a woefully low priority.

Because, in advanced old age, the progression of many diseases like dementia or cancer means constant deterioration and finally death, 'there's nothing more that we can do' often gives rise to a kind of therapeutic nihilism. This overlooks the fact that real improvement in quality of life is definitely possible during the last years or months of life.

The most important means of maintaining quality of life in old age is human contact. This should not be underestimated when the question arises of how old people can be protected from spiritual and sensory deprivation. The importance of contact can be seen from the fact that sensory deprivation can lead to faulty perception. Delusions, auto-stimulation by screaming, shouting, knocking on the wall with mobility aids, or even self-harm by scratching the skin, are alarm signals for spiritual and sensory deprivation.

Contact, then, is an essential contribution to the wellbeing of old people – especially those who are seriously ill. To prevent sensory deprivation there is need of physical contact. This is where the Shōnishin acupuncturist has a part to play, as in Shōnishin he has a proven means of sensory stimulation.

10.3 Energetic regression

As mentioned elsewhere in this book, in certain situations we can all draw, at any time, on old energetic patterns that have been laid down as a resource. Young people and adults have access to the three families, the six *keiraku* and the five phases; kindergarten children have the three families to draw on.

Very old people are also able to draw on old resources. As the motor, sensory and energetic aspects of being are closely interlinked, in parallel with the loss of motor and sensory capacities there is also a loss of energetic potential. The evidence seems to suggest that an energetic retrogression takes place. Not only does the subject-matter of the *keiraku* and the three families come back into the foreground at this stage of life; the weakening meridians also form a unity, just like the immature meridians following birth.

This being so, in old people who are the most seriously ill or immobile there is little point in treating individual meridians. On the contrary, the meridians should be treated in their 'family constellation', and here the issues of the front family come first: being uprooted, difficulties with nutrition and digestion, loss of contact, weakening immunity, respiratory problems – to name a few 'front family' themes. We can see that the big challenges for very old people are the same as they are for a baby. These challenges at the beginning and end of life are:

- How do I get nourished?

- How do I move with gravity?

- How do I breathe?

- How do I get support from the outside world?

- How reliable is this?

- Am I still worthy of attention?

In keeping with the dominance of the front family, treatment is performed as in the the basic treatment. This can be limited to areas on the forearm and lower leg through which the front family meridians run. The strength of touch for the stroking technique is also the same as it is for treating a baby. The rate of stroking, in contrast to what it should be for adults, is well below 120 strokes per minute.

11

Treatment at Home

Parents ask me all the time whether they can do Shōnishin at home. One possibility is to show them specific stimulation techniques I have devised, based on Shonishin, which they can do with a table-tennis ball or massage ball. Then the parents have a simple, straightforward treatment technique that is suitable for use at home.

Depending on the age of the child, treatment can be done when changing a nappy, as part of a bedtime ritual, or after nursery/kindergarten or school. In acute cases treatment can be given in between appointments and treatment done by the Shōnishin acupuncturist can be supported by the parents in a meaningful way, on their own authority, at home. Involving the parents in a system that supports development or therapy also leads to greater confidence when dealing with their children's disorders or illnesses, and this too can have a beneficial effect on their children's health.

11.1 Conditions for treatment at home

For doing treatment parents need only a table-tennis ball, a small, soft massage ball about 6cm in diameter, and kitchen weighing scales. Depending what symptoms or needs the child has, either gentle or vigorous stimulation can be used. The table-tennis ball is suited to gentle stimulation; vigorous stimulation is best done with the massage ball. Babies should be treated only with a table-tennis ball.

How to do treatment with a ball: instructions for parents from the Shōnishin acupuncturist

- The right way of handling the ball

- The right pressure

- The rate of repetition for the rolling procedure

THE RIGHT WAY OF HANDLING THE BALL

- Table-tennis ball – make your hand into the shape of a small dish to contain the ball (Figure 11.1).

- Hedgehog ball – place your hand flat on top of the ball.

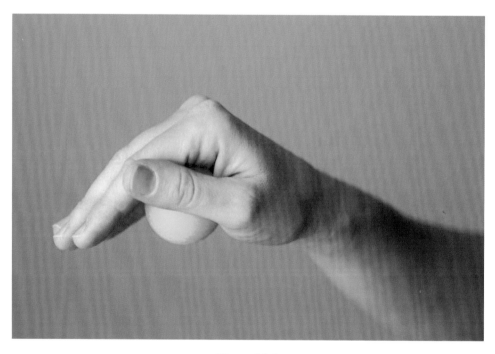

Figure 11.1

THE RIGHT PRESSURE

Treatment with the massage ball can be done with three different degrees of pressure. The parents need kitchen weighing scales in order to try out and practise the appropriate degree of pressure. The following figures in grams are (lowest value) for toddlers and (highest value) for children older than 6 years. Intermediate ages fall between the lowest and the highest value.

Table 11.1: Pressure in grams

	Pressure (grams)
Light pressure	50–150 (babies: 20–50)
Moderate pressure	400–700
Strong pressure	1000–1500

When doing treatment with the table-tennis ball, only light pressure is used.

THE RATE OF REPETITION FOR THE ROLLING PROCEDURE

How many times the rolling is repeated depends on:

- whether you are using the table-tennis ball or the massage ball
- the degree of pressure you are using
- how old the child is.

Babies should be treated only with the table-tennis ball.

Table 11.2: Rate of repetition for the rolling procedure

	Age	Light pressure	Moderate pressure	Strong pressure
Table-tennis ball	1–3 months	3x		
	3–12 months	5x		
	> 12 months	5–8x		
Hedgehog ball	1–3 years	3x	3–5x	3–5x
	4–7 years	5x	5–8x	5–9x
	8–12 years	8x	8–10x	9–10x

When parents should not treat their child

Treatment should not be done:

- if the child has a temperature

- during the first three days following a vaccination

- if there is uncertainty about the child's condition

- if the child refuses treatment.

11.2 Home treatment information sheets for parents

The following information sheets for parents with treatment examples can be downloaded from www.singingdragon.com/catalogue/9781848191600/resources. The practitioner treating the child should fill in:

- Practice/name of the practitioner

- Number of treatments per day or per week to be done by the parents at home

- Name of the child

- Rate of repetition of the rolling procedure, as applicable to the part of the body concerned

- Pressure (in grams) with which the ball should be rolled over the body for the child concerned

Finally, the information sheet can be given out to parents. When this is added to information given by the practitioner, the parents will have helpful support for doing the treatment at home.

The first information sheet deals with treatment of babies. In principle, home treatment of a baby is done exclusively with the table-tennis ball and with 'light' pressure. Regardless of the reason for treatment, babies are massaged by their parents according to a standardised procedure (see information sheet).

This treatment supports in particular:

- a baby's development

- her immune system

- her regulation (sleep/wake rhythm, digestion, startle response, muscle tone)

- a restless baby

- a baby who is teething.

In other words, by treating their baby at home, harassed parents are putting the baby, and ultimately themselves, in a good mood.

The following information sheets for parents are provided:

- Home treatment information sheet 1: Babies

- Home treatment information sheet 2: Lack of Appetite

- Home treatment information sheet 3: Asthma/Bronchitis/Cough

- Home treatment information sheet 4: Bedwetting

- Home treatment information sheet 5: Problems Falling Asleep

- Home treatment information sheet 6: Sleep Disturbance/Crying at Night

- Home treatment information sheet 7: Susceptibility to Infection

- Home treatment information sheet 8: Neurodermatitis

- Home treatment information sheet 9: Constipation/Diarrhoea

Home treatment information sheet example: Asthma in a 4-year-old Child

In the following example, entries by the Shōnishin acupuncturist are shown in red. To assist comprehension I have added illustrations (Figures 11.2–11.8) to the treatment example; these are referred to in the text.

Home treatment information sheet example
Asthma in a 4-year-old Child

Given out by (practice/practitioner): Joe Bloggs

Recommended treatment: 1 x per day/(per week) for Lydia M.

Dear parents,

With these recommendations for treatment at home you will be supporting the therapy your child is receiving from me. Please proceed as described below.

You will need: A hedgehog ball.

1. Using moderate pressure, starting next to the 7th (prominent) neck vertebra, roll the hedgehog ball towards the shoulder joint (Figure 11.2).

    Repeat: 5 x (first on one shoulder, then the other).

    Pressure: approx. 500 grams.

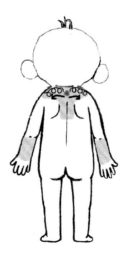

2.   Then, with light pressure, roll over the area alongside the thoracic spine, from the 7th neck vertebra down to level with the lower tip of the shoulder blade (Figure 11.3).

Repeat: 5 x.

Pressure: approx. 100 grams.

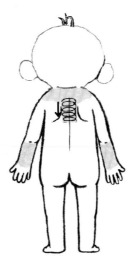

3.   Then, with light pressure, roll over the outside of both forearms, from the elbows to the wrists (Figure 11.4).

Repeat: 5 x.

Pressure: approx. 100 grams.

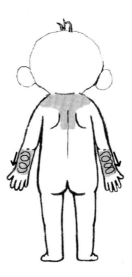

4. With the same pressure, roll over the inside of both forearms, from the elbows to the wrists (Figure 11.5).

    Repeat: 5 x.

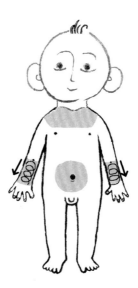

5. Continue the treatment, rolling with light pressure from the top of the breastbone to the shoulder joints (below the collarbones) (Figure 11.6).

    Repeat: 5 x on both sides.

    Pressure: approx. 100 grams.

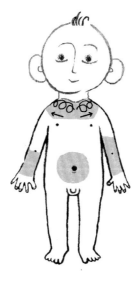

6. Finally, with light pressure roll clockwise around the navel (Figure 11.7 and 11.8).

Repeat: 5 x.

Pressure: approx. 100 grams.

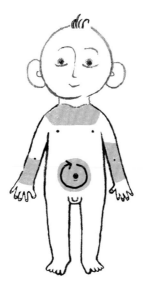

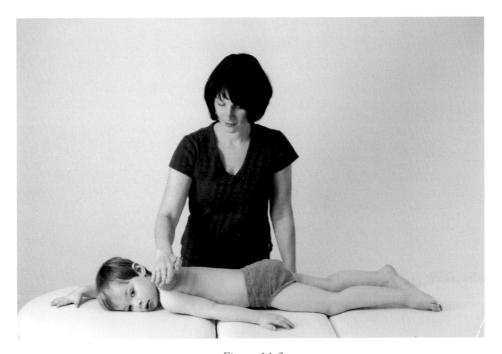

Figure 11.2

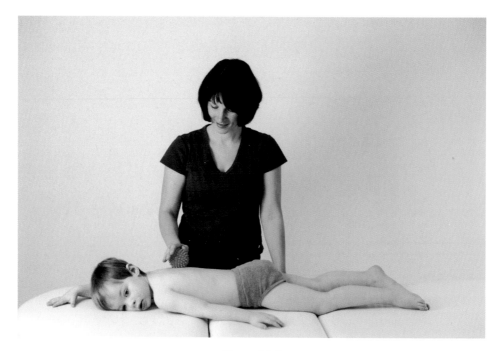

Figure 11.3

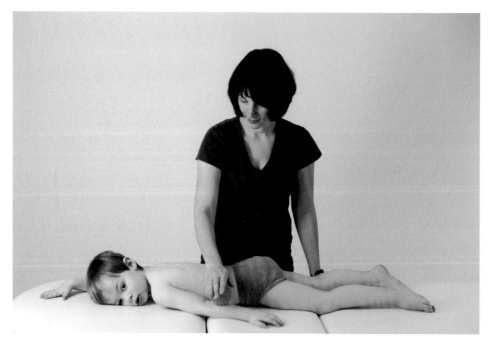

Figure 11.4

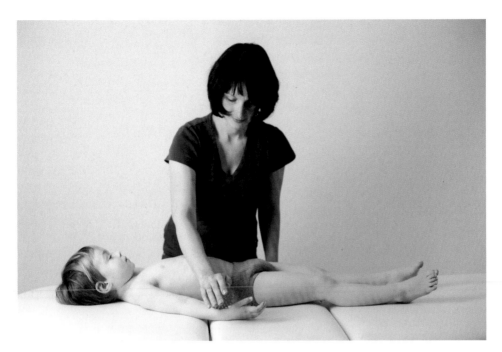

Figure 11.5

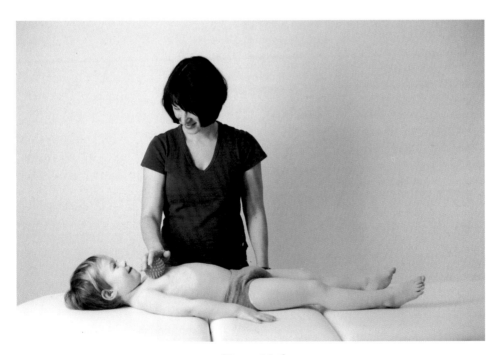

Figure 11.6

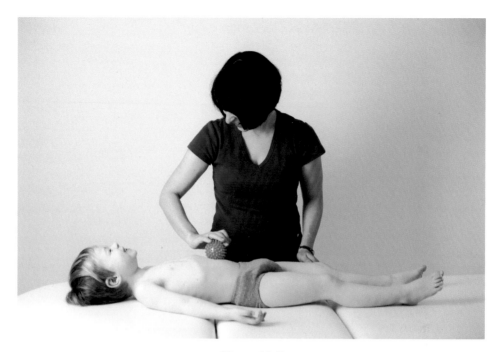

Figure 11.7

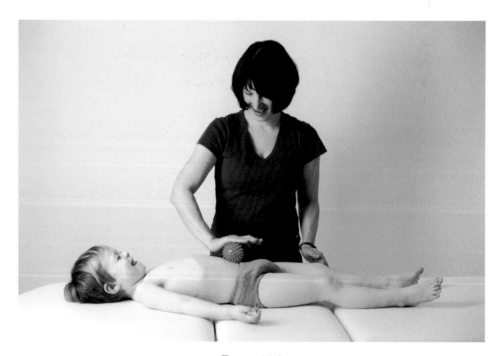

Figure 11.8

Home treatment information sheet 1

Babies

Given out by (practice/practitioner): _____

Recommended treatment: _____ x per day/per week for _____.

Dear parents,

With these recommendations for treatment at home you will be supporting the therapy your child is receiving from me. Please proceed as described below.

You will need: A table-tennis ball.

Pressure: _____ grams.

1. First, put your baby down on his/her tummy. Roll the table-tennis ball along the spine from top to bottom, beginning each time from the (prominent) 7th vertebra and finishing over the sacrum.

    Repeat: _____ x.

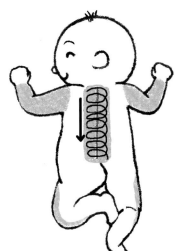

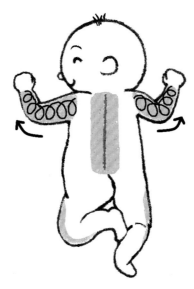

2. Then roll over the outside of the arm, beginning from the shoulder joint, down to the wrist, first on one arm, then the other. Your baby can stay on his/her tummy or lie on his/her back.

    Repeat: _____ x on each arm.

3. Leg treatment is done in the same way as for the arm: first down the front of one leg from the hip joint to the ankle, then the other leg.

    Repeat: _____ x on each leg.

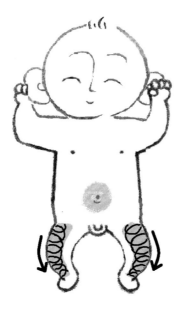

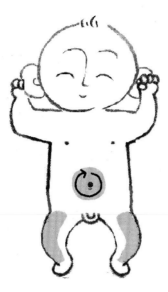

4. Finally, roll clockwise around the navel.

Repeat: _____ x.

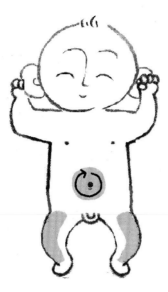

Home treatment information sheet 2

Loss of Appetite

Given out by (practice/practitioner): _____

Recommended treatment: _____ x per day/per week for _____.

Dear parents,

With these recommendations for treatment at home you will be supporting the therapy your child is receiving from me. Please proceed as described below.

   You will need: A hedgehog ball.

1.   Roll with light pressure clockwise around the navel.

      Repeat: _____ x.

      Pressure: _____ grams.

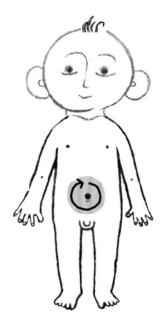

2. Then with moderate pressure roll over the area between the shoulder blades and the thoracic spine, down as far as the waist.

    Repeat: _____ x on each side, beginning at the top every time.

    Pressure: _____ grams.

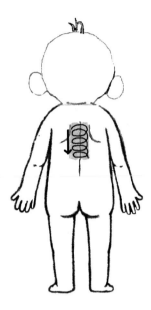

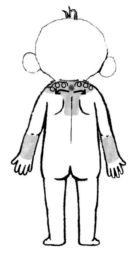

Home treatment information sheet 3

Asthma/Bronchitis/Cough

Given out by (practice/practitioner): _____

Recommended treatment: _____ x per day/per week for _____.

Dear parents,

With these recommendations for treatment at home you will be supporting the therapy your child is receiving from me. Please proceed as described below.

　You will need: A hedgehog ball.

1.　Starting next to the 7th (prominent) vertebra, roll the hedgehog ball with moderate pressure towards the shoulder joint.

　　Repeat: _____ x (first on one shoulder, then the other).

　　Pressure: _____ grams.

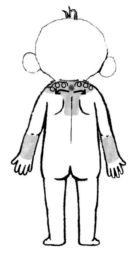

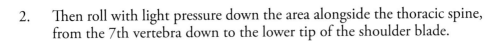

2. Then roll with light pressure down the area alongside the thoracic spine, from the 7th vertebra down to the lower tip of the shoulder blade.

Repeat: _____ x.

Pressure: _____ grams.

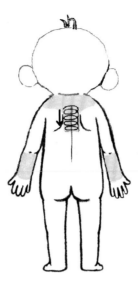

3. Then roll with light pressure along the outside of the forearms, from the elbow to the wrist.

Repeat: _____ x.

Pressure: _____ grams.

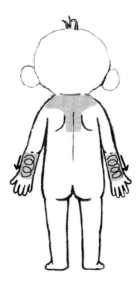

4. Roll with the same pressure over the inside of both forearms, from the elbow to the wrist.

Repeat: _____ x.

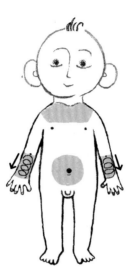

5. Continue the treatment with light pressure from the top of the breastbone towards the shoulder joint (below the collarbone).

Repeat: _____ x on each side.

Pressure: _____ grams.

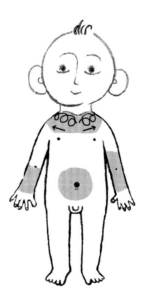

6.   Finally, roll with light pressure clockwise around the navel.

Repeat: _____ x.

Pressure: _____ grams.

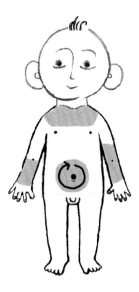

Bedwetting

Given out by (practice/practitioner): _____

Recommended treatment: _____ x per day/per week for _____.

Dear parents,

With these recommendations for treatment at home you will be supporting the therapy your child is receiving from me. Please proceed as described below.

    You will need: A hedgehog ball.

1.   Your child is lying on his/her back. With moderate pressure roll the hedgehog ball clockwise above the pubic bone.

    Repeat: _____ x.

    Pressure: _____ grams.

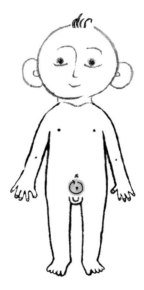

2. Next, with your child lying on his/her tummy, roll with moderate pressure down the area alongside the lumbar spine, from the waist down to the sacrum.

    Repeat: _____ x.

    Pressure: _____ grams.

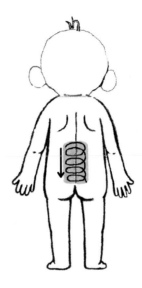

3. Then, with strong pressure, roll clockwise on the sacrum.

    Repeat: _____ x.

    Pressure: _____ grams.

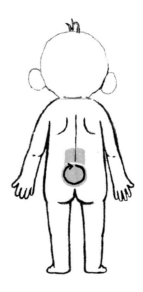

Problems Falling Asleep

Given out by (practice/practitioner): _____

Recommended treatment: _____ x per day/per week for _____.

Dear parents,

With these recommendations for treatment at home you will be supporting the therapy your child is receiving from me. Please proceed as described below

    You will need: A hedgehog ball.

1.   Your child is lying on his/her tummy. Beginning at the shoulder joint, roll the hedgehog ball with strong pressure above the top of the shoulder blade towards the spine, and between the spine and the shoulder blade down to the tip of the shoulder blade.

    Repeat: _____ x on each side.

    Pressure: _____ grams.

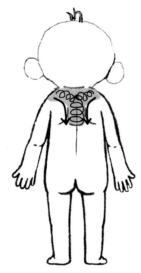

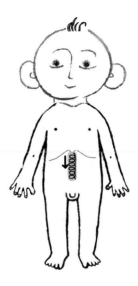

2. Then, with your child lying on his/her back, roll the hedgehog ball with light pressure over the upper abdominal area, from the tip of the breastbone to the navel.

Repeat: _____ x.

Pressure: _____ grams.

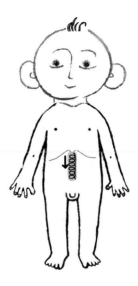

Home treatment information sheet 6

Sleep Disturbance/Crying at Night

Given out by (practice/practitioner): _____

Recommended treatment: _____ x per day/per week for _____.

Dear parents,

With these recommendations for treatment at home you will be supporting the therapy your child is receiving from me. Please proceed as described below.

You will need: A hedgehog ball.

1.   Your child is lying on his/her tummy. Beginning at the shoulder joint, roll the hedgehog ball with strong pressure above the top of the shoulder blade towards the spine, and between the spine and the shoulder blade down to the tip of the shoulder blade.

Repeat: _____ x on each side.

Pressure: _____ grams.

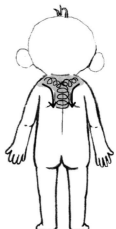

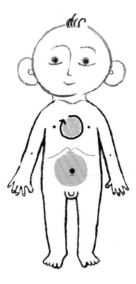

2. Then, with your child on his/her back, roll the hedgehog ball with light pressure clockwise over the chest, level with the nipples.

   Repeat: _____ x.

   Pressure: _____ grams.

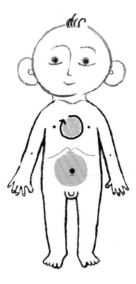

3. Likewise, with the same pressure, roll over the upper abdomen from the tip of the breastbone to below the navel.

   Repeat: _____ x.

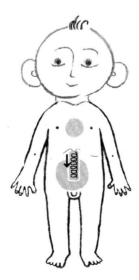

4.   Finally, with the same pressure, roll clockwise around the navel.

Repeat: _____ x.

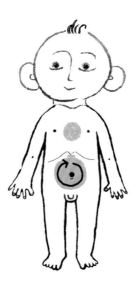

Susceptibility to Infection

Given out by (practice/practitioner): _____

Recommended treatment: _____ x per day/per week for _____.

Dear parents,

With these recommendations for treatment at home you will be supporting the therapy your child is receiving from me. Please proceed as described below.

You will need: A hedgehog ball.

1. Starting next to the 7th (prominent) vertebra, roll the hedgehog ball with moderate pressure towards the shoulder joint.

    Repeat: _____ x (first one shoulder, then the other).

    Pressure: _____ grams.

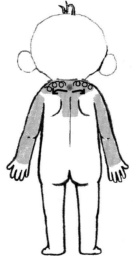

2. Then roll with light pressure alongside the thoracic spine, from the 7th vertebra down to the tip of the shoulder blade.

Repeat: _____ x.

Pressure: _____ grams.

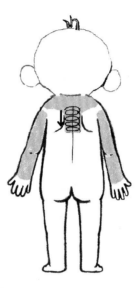

3. Then roll with light pressure down the inside of the forearms, from the shoulder joint to the wrist.

Repeat: _____ x.

Pressure: _____ grams.

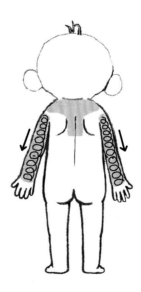

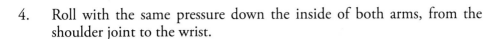

4. Roll with the same pressure down the inside of both arms, from the shoulder joint to the wrist.

    Repeat: _____ x.

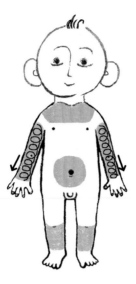

5. Continue the treatment with light pressure from the top of the breastbone towards the shoulder joint (below the collarbone).

    Repeat: _____ x on each side.

    Pressure: _____ grams.

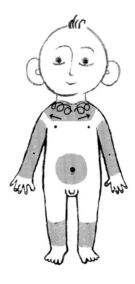

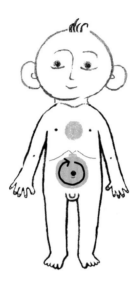

6.   Finally, roll with light pressure clockwise around the navel.

Repeat: _____ x.

Pressure: ____ grams.

Neurodermatitis

Given out by (practice/practitioner): _____

Recommended treatment: _____ x per day/per week for _____.

Dear parents,

With these recommendations for treatment at home you will be supporting the therapy your child is receiving from me. Please proceed as described below.

You will need: A hedgehog ball.

1. Roll with light pressure clockwise around the navel.

    Repeat: _____ x.

    Pressure: ____ grams.

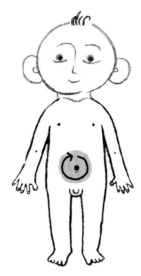

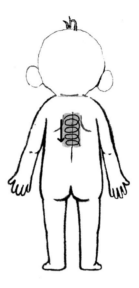

2. Then roll with moderate pressure over the area between the shoulder blades and the thoracic spine, down to waist level.

Repeat: _____ x.

Pressure: _____ grams.

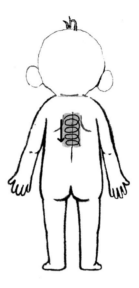

Home treatment information sheet 9

Constipation/Diarrhoea

Given out by (practice/practitioner): _____

Recommended treatment: _____ x per day/per week for _____.

Dear parents,

With these recommendations for treatment at home you will be supporting the therapy your child is receiving from me. Please proceed as described below.

You will need: A hedgehog ball.

1. Roll with light pressure around the navel (clockwise for constipation; anti-clockwise for diarrhoea).

    Repeat: _____ x.

    Pressure: _____ grams.

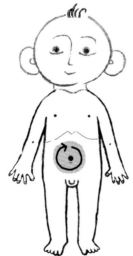

2. Your child is now lying on his/her tummy.

a. Constipation: Roll with strong pressure over the area immediately above the pelvic crest, from the outside towards the centre (i.e. the sacrum), first on one side, then the other.

Repeat: _____ x (from the outside towards the centre each time).

Pressure: _____ grams.

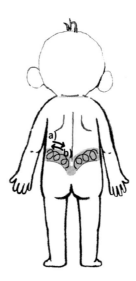

b. Diarrhoea: Roll with moderate pressure over the area immediately above the pelvic crest, from the centre towards the outside – first on one side, then the other.

Repeat: _____ x (from the inside towards the outside each time).

Pressure: _____ grams.

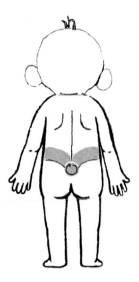

3. Finally, roll with moderate pressure clockwise over the sacrum.

    Repeat: _____ x.

    Pressure: _____ grams.

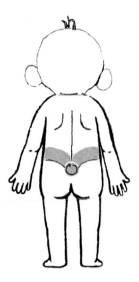

12

Examples from Practice

The case studies presented here have been kindly provided by colleagues from Germany, Austria, Switzerland, Italy and Mexico, whom I have trained in recent years. They illustrate the broad compass of Shōnishin treatment.

The following case studies have been selected to show a representative sample of treatment with Shōnishin. Of course, I also have case studies in which Shōnishin treatment was not successful. Ultimately we are concerned here not with a panacea but with a method which, like any other, has its strong and weak points. The essential strength of Shōnishin lies in its suitability for treating children, which has led to its exceptionally high degree of acceptability among children and their parents.

12.1 Case studies – Babies

Diagnoses

- Three-month colic

- Sleep disturbance at night

- Excessive crying

- Severe hypo-ischaemic brain damage

To begin with the youngest ones – the commonest complaints they have to contend with in the first months after birth are caused by digestive problems. So it was with Miriam – as the following study shows.

Three-month colic

Miriam, 6 weeks

Recorded by A.H., Shiatsu practitioner in Switzerland

For the past two weeks I have been treating a 6-week-old baby who is suffering every day from stomach cramps and wind. She appears to be in a fair bit of pain, keeps pulling her legs in, and is then very restless.

So far I have done three treatments (basic treatment, vibration treatment of the front family source points) and on each occasion she has had a day without cramps, on the last occasion even three days, she is sleeping better and her digestion has been stimulated.

Digestive problems are certainly not pleasant for the baby, but sleep problems can really drive parents round the bend.

Sleep disturbance at night

Lena, 3 months

Recorded by Dr I.W., consultant in anaesthesia and intensive care in Austria

Lena is the daughter of someone I know. She cries every evening as soon as she is put to bed. During the day she is an easy, contented baby, has no sleep problems, is exclusively breastfed, digestion is normal. Paediatrician says 'everything is OK'. The parents are under great nervous strain from lack of sleep. Lena won't go to bed at night, often has to be carried, driven or rocked for hours until finally, mostly after midnight, she falls asleep.

03.07.2012: On an evening visit to Lena's family I tried Shōnishin (basic treatment). Lena was then put to bed and straightaway fell asleep!

Repeated treatment on 06.07. and 11.07. Since then Lena has been going to sleep without crying and her parents are having even more enjoyment with her.

Excessive crying will sooner or later drive parents to the limit. To my knowledge there is no method as effective as Shōnishin for treating babies who cry excessively – a blessing for parents and children.

Excessive crying
Vivien, 4 months

> Recorded by Dr S.I., consultant in physical medicine in Germany
>
> Vivien's mother told me about her child's attacks of crying that could last as long as four or five hours in the evening and at night-time, as well as restlessness and breastfeeding problems.
>
> In my osteopathy/manual therapy examination I found, and treated, functional disorders in the suboccipital area. Functional disorders like this are often the cause of attacks of crying and restlessness. With Vivien, unfortunately, this was not the case. She continued to be very restless, waking up to 10 times during the night, and often had crying fits for no reason during the day.
>
> Then I started treating her with Shōnishin. After the first treatment her mother told me that Vivien was already much calmer and sleeping better. After four sessions Vivien was able to sleep through the night and was much more relaxed during the day. Her mother says that her whole being has changed for the better with Shōnishin.

When treating children with severe disabilities, you have to think of progress in terms of steps measured 'by the millimetre'. It is always helpful to complement these children's treatment with Shōnishin.

Severe hypoxic-ischaemic brain damage
Florian, 8½ months

> Recorded by occupational therapist and complementary therapist D.J. in Germany
>
> *Reason for treatment*: Following peripartum asphyxia, following seizures; persistent cholestatic hepatopathy, nephrocalcinosis, incipient spastic-dystonic motor disorder.
>
> *Date of birth*: 24.02.2011. Home birth in the 39th week after 50 hours in labour (110 minutes contractions). Additional problems breastfeeding. Admitted to local hospital after six days.

Condition on admission: Severe reduction in general condition, apathy, hypotonia, peripherally cold. Reduced skin turgor. Pronounced jaundice of skin and sclerae, rhythmic spasms/clonus in the right hand and foot, alternating tonic extension/flaccid.

Case history: In addition to initial diagnoses, the following were observed during the time following birth: Opisthotonus (hyperextension), lopsidedness, head turned predominantly to the right, gaze predominantly to the left; following birth, a large cephalo-haematoma on the upper right side of the head; since September, strong spasms, especially in the arms; he has had two hernias already (one on each side).

Therapies: Eye clinic, osteopathy, physiotherapy, curative education, baby swimming.

Progression of treatment: Florian has had four appointments with me. At the first appointment he appeared very congested, had an unstable gaze and seemed abstracted and stressed. He had a fungal infection on his legs (lateral on the right, anterior and dorsal on the left). His mouth was permanently open, with a lot of thick saliva.

4.11. Shōnishin – Basic treatment + needle held on Du Mai 14 (distinct reddening around Du Mai 14). Then cried hard, and mucus immediately reduced. Report following treatment: He cried a lot, and the next day had a raised temperature (up to 39.4°C). His temperature remains high, approx. 37.8°C. His gaze is more alert.

8.11. Basic treatment + vibration on Ki 1, Pc 5, Pc 7; also LI 4 + Li 3; needle held on Du Mai 14. Following treatment Florian sleeps a lot, and soundly. He seems relaxed, his gaze is clearer, his eyes bright. He has had no more fits since the first treatment. Still having spasms. The parents report sensitivity to wind.

11.11. Basic treatment; Li 4 and LI 3; Du 14 (holding the needle); Ki 1, Pc 5, Pc 7; Gb 37. During treatment Florian smiles and is much more relaxed than previously. He also makes more eye contact.

15.11. The parents report that he perceives more, is more responsive, happier, and reaching out for things more. His eyes are moving further to the right. After the last treatment he again had a raised temperature; his temperature is now lower all the time (37.1°C to 37.2°C).

12.2 Case studies – Toddlers

Diagnoses

- Neurodermatitis

- Behavioural problems

- No specific cause

- Epilepsy

Treating toddlers is often challenging, not only for Shōnishin acupuncturists but also for paediatricians, physiotherapists, occupational therapists and others. At this age most children are more or less clearly at the 'defiant stage'. Their action is set in 'refusal mode' and the most important word is 'No!' A respectful but definite manner can be an advantage. It is pointless to carry out an examination or treatment if the child resists, which would also forfeit a lot of trust on the part of the child.

As a Shōnishin acupuncturist it is important to be clear that Shōnishin is not done as a lifesaving therapy. If a child doesn't want to be treated at any cost, then put it off until another time.

The following example is that of a boy with neurodermatitis. This involves a skin dysregulation that has increased markedly in recent decades. In most cases neurodermatitis appears in children aged 1 and over – a torment for the child and parents.

Neurodermatitis

Boy, 20 months

Recorded by Professor R.W., MD, Department of General Paediatrics and Adolescent Medicine, Division of Neonatology in Austria

Boy aged 20 months, atopic dermatitis since the age of 3 months, twice at the age of 4 months; six months of cortisone treatment on the face. Currently, with basic care, intermittent mild skin lesions especially on the wrists and lower legs laterally. If the care regime was omitted for one day, the next day there would be distinct worsening of the condition, with newly affected patches approx. 2cm in diameter. After bathing (2x weekly; with skin medication), severe reddening for two days.

In the 'neurodermatitis area' (reaction zone according to Tanioka) on the back there is altered skin similar to 'goosebumps' (since the age of 11 months).

Mild skin changes (neurodermatitis) on the wrist, elbow and lower leg (red, dry). No itching.

So far I have done three basic treatments, and one very gentle tapping technique on the 'neurodermatitis area' on the back – from the top downwards, and from lateral to medial. Since then the 'goosebumps' on the 'neurodermatitis area' on the back have completely disappeared, the skin is much improved, basic care is being continued, when there is intermittent omission of basic care there is no occurrence of newly affected patches. Frequent 'splashing around' in water, even without medication, no longer leads to deterioration.

The next example describes a case from my own practice, one that I frequently encounter. At the toddler stage a child with a temperature can be thrown off centre by the recurrence of feverish nightmares – often the cause of sleep disturbance.

Behavioural problems (with sleep disturbance, general eczema)
Philipp B., 16 months

Shortly before Christmas 2006 Philipp had a fever; for four days his temperature was above 41°C. He was given antibiotics, which disagreed with him; he had vomiting and a rash erupted all over his body.

Since that time (four weeks before) everything had been 'out of kilter': he was suffering from severe sleep disturbance, so that his mother was having to go to his room up to 30 times during the night. If she didn't go to him, then he would react with what she described as 'hysterics' and bang his head against objects, floor or wall so hard that his forehead was covered in bruises. In addition, since then he had developed such enormous separation anxiety that during the day it was impossible for his mother to leave him on his own, even for a moment – even when going to the toilet she had to carry him with her, otherwise he would have hysterics.

Regarding previous history, apart from the fact that birth was normal, and so was early development, it is worth mentioning that Philipp was a crooked baby. Twice he had osteopathic treatment for this. Moreover, he could already walk by himself at the age of 10½ months. On examination he was found to have had papular eczema, which was spread all over his body (for the previous four weeks). The 'light' cortisone cream with which Philipp was occasionally treated led to a temporary improvement in his skin condition, but never to completely clear skin.

Treatment and progression: As there had been nothing abnormal in Philipp up to the age of 14 months and his severe sleep disturbance, separation anxiety and eczema were linked to a feverish illness, it made sense to assume that the fever (four days above 41°C!) had thrown him off centre, with the corresponding psychic and organic reaction. Therefore basic treatment and meridian treatment of the front family circuits were carried out in order to bring him back to his centre.

I treated him twice a week with basic treatment and front family meridian treatment, including yuan points – four times to begin with. At the first appointment Philipp would only let me treat him sitting on his mother's lap, with plenty of distraction. At the second appointment his mother said that the day before he had had such a violent tantrum that he had banged his head until his forehead bled. This treatment was also done with him sitting on his mother's lap.

Four days later, at the third appointment, Philipp let me treat him sitting next to his mother on the therapy table. She said that for the past two nights he had woken up only once during the night. His skin seemed to be settling down; the eczema on his trunk was scarcely visible any more; there were clear signs of eczema only on both his forearms and hands.

Up to the fourth session there was no change – continuing sound sleep, the skin seemed to be stabilising, but tantrums were occurring as often as before, especially if his mother didn't give in to his demands to be carried around. So I decided to change my treatment strategy. His behaviour showed me that the lateral family also needed some support. Philipp's tantrums were escalating to the point that it was very difficult for him to return to his centre (front family). Therefore, after stabilising the front family, the interchange between the front and lateral families needed strengthening. So for the next two sessions I treated the lateral family.

At the sixth treatment his mother said that Philipp was not yet free of tantrums, but they were less frequent, and she thought it was really important to tell me that he would clearly calm down more easily. So we decided on an interval of two months before further treatment.

In the course of those two months there were two violent 'attacks' when Philipp banged his head sore; otherwise the nights were peaceful, he would occasionally wake up once. His skin was free of lesions, except for a small, sore, red rash on his right forearm and the base of his right thumb. We agreed to continue with Shōnishin treatments once every two weeks. I treated the front family. Two weeks after the third session we agreed that there was no need for further treatment. His skin was stable, separation anxiety no longer appeared to be a problem, and his tantrums had reduced to 'normal' for a 20-month-old child.

The next case study shows a Shōnishin acupuncturist treating a toddler with great sensitivity. The respectful way in which she approaches the child and limits the treatment to the bare essentials are key to successful rapport-building and treatment.

No specific cause
Eva, nearly 2 years old

Recorded by Shiatsu practitioner A.S. in Austria

Eva is a friend's daughter. There is nothing obvious the matter with her, so for me this was just an opportunity to try out Shōnishin with toddlers.

Eva will be 2 in August. The birth was without complications (her brother, aged 5, came into the world by Caesarean section). She had a brief crawling phase – she wanted to walk straightaway. To begin with, her brother was a bit jealous, but since she has become OK as a playmate they have been a good team, with occasional squabbles when Matthias (her brother) sets the boundaries and she often makes her feelings known by crying – not for long, but very dramatically. (Mother says that now and then she can be a bit of a drama queen.)

Eva seems very independent and is not watched all the time. Her physique is sturdy, without being fat. Her mother finds her very easy and Eva is allowed to spend a lot of time trying out different things.

What I find fascinating is that she always looks things over very carefully before using them. Her mother says she's really looking forward to painting and making things with Eva, because she is already showing a great deal of interest in in such things – unlike Matthias. Eva also looks for a long time at people she doesn't know – she has a searching look, and sometimes she hides behind her mother for a little while. Her expression is quite different when she smiles – from rather dark to very bright and warm.

Eva didn't want to lie down for Shōnishin treatment, and she was also a bit shy. The video of Masanori Tanioka and his playful way of relating to children has helped me a lot. After playing with Eva for a little while, her mum took her onto her lap, and I started working on Mum – then simply transferred my attention to Eva (I asked first; no answer – neither 'yes' nor 'no' – just a searching look). She became very still, as if listening on the inside.

I stuck to the basic treatment without tapping or vibration techniques. Then Eva's attitude towards me changed completely – I was to read to her, and she showed me various toys.

The second time I did much the same, and it was much easier. Again, Eva became very still. I observed a lot of tension in her legs and abdomen, her back was soft and fluid, her shoulders seemed a bit feeble.

The third time I caught her during a nappy change, and so I was able to treat her lying down, which is much easier. Again, she grew quite still and thoughtful. Her eyes take on a distant look.

In all three treatments I stuck to the basic treatment without tapping or vibration techniques, as no real material came to light. Her mother observed that on treatment days Eva was very calm.

One Shōnishin acupuncturist recorded her experience of doing Shōnishin with her own son, who had a serious diagnosis. It is interesting to see how positive her outlook on life must be – the way she describes her son's small steps forward is a source of encouragement for anyone with a burden to carry.

Epilepsy
Lenny, 2½ years

Recorded by I.K., Shiatsu practitioner in Austria

My son Lenny was born on 5.11.2009; he is my third child. The pregnancy was fine, the birth quick and spontaneous, three days before the date reckoned. On the third day we were discharged, and quite content. Lenny slept a lot; it was difficult to wake him for a feed, and after the meconium he passed no stools for ten days. On day 7 the seizures started, later diagnosed as BNS epilepsy. Despite a long stay in hospital, ACTH treatment, and later ketogenic diet, we couldn't get a grip on the seizures. After a change of medication he was having attacks for six months. Now he's had no attacks for 21 months.

Lenny's development is delayed. He prefers lying on his back, reaches for toys, brings his hands to the centre and crosses the centre. He's not interested in his feet. In contrast to his first year, he has flaccid muscle tone. He rolls onto his tummy, but doesn't like to stay like that. He has difficulty leaning on his arms. He also rolls from his tummy back onto his back, but doesn't move around very far in space. He can sit only with support. His legs won't take any weight.

Since Lenny has stopped having seizures, he hasn't been on a ketogenic diet any more. Now he enjoys his food and likes almost anything. Sometimes he doesn't chew very well, and then he chokes. His tongue doesn't move very much and he doesn't stick it out. No language development. His eyes were weak to begin with (i.e. he couldn't fix his eyes on things). But his hearing has been good from the start. He is very calm and a relaxed, contented child. Likes music, and now also likes watching his siblings.

Treatment: I began with the basic treatment, plus tapping around the navel. For the next three days I also did the front family and the corresponding yuan points. There was an improvement in his grip; hand movement grew steadier.

The next week I concentrated on the back family. One of my aims was for Lenny to make progress with language and standing up. I did the treatment again on three successive days. Then a break.

I was surprised one day when Lenny tried to get up onto his feet. First I grasped his knees and showed him how to stretch them out, then, with me holding him only by the pelvis, he was standing up by himself, making rowing movements with his arms and having fun with that.

It also struck us that he was more alert, quicker in his reactions and very interested in language. He had also enjoyed watching us talk previously, and his tongue became more mobile.

Since then he has been having a Shōnishin treatment every ten days. His early learning therapist, ophthalmologist and physiotherapist are admiring Lenny's progress and sharing our joy.

12.3 Case studies – 3–5-year-olds

Diagnoses

- Otitis media
- Susceptibility to infection
- Sleep disturbance
- Behavioural problems

At kindergarten or school, abnormalities relating to movement and behaviour can be spotted, as the teachers are able to observe the children over a long period of time, and also to compare them with children of the same age.

In the case below the topic is the frequently observed link between chronic inflammation of the middle ear and abnormal language development. Children with delayed speech and/or language development are often not spotted until they are at kindergarten or school, because this is the first time they are outside the home environment and part of a new social group. At home there is often 'group blindness' – speech and language deficits are less obvious within the 'family team'.

Otitis media (chronically recurring); language disorder
Guillermo, 3 years

Recorded by Dr L.R., paediatrician in Mexico

Case history: Guillermo is soon to have tonsil surgery, as he is very susceptible to infection. Respiratory tract infections go straight to his ear. He has inflammation of the middle ear at least once a month and this has been going on for over a year. It is treated every time with antibiotics, cortisone nasal spray, antihistamines and paracetamol. His parents want to have one last try with alternative therapy before surgical intervention.

Guillermo, the second child, was delivered by planned Caesarean section. The pregnancy was normal. Guillermo did everything a bit 'later' than his sister (said his mother). He couldn't hold his head up until 5 months, or sit by himself until 8 months, crawled at 12 months and walked at 18 months.

His ear problems began in his first year. Chronic, undiagnosed *otitis media* presumably led to a hearing problem, and hence a speech disorder too. For this reason Guillermo has been having speech therapy since the age of 2½, but he still cannot express himself clearly. Guillermo often has tantrums, is irritable all the time, cries easily and gets into his parents' bed every night, as he says that he is scared and having nightmares. His mother also mentioned that Guillermo eats very little, and reluctantly.

Examination: On physical examination posture was hypotonic, the head rather large in relation to the body, the skin pallid, yellowish and dry, very red tongue. During examination there were no other abnormalities.

Treatment: Altogether I have done six treatments, one a week.

> Basic treatment: point treatment on the following acupuncture points: LI 4, LI 11, Li 3, He 5, Lu 9, Bl 20, Bl 23, St 36.

> For acute *otitis*: basic treatment and point treatment (SI 14, LI 4, LI 11, Gb 41, SJ 5).

Progress: At the first consultation I did only the basic treatment. The second time (one week later) Guillermo arrived with acute *otitis media* and severe earache. His mother said she had not observed any change, so I did point treatment as well.

After the fifth session he had a slight cold, but this time without a high temperature and also without ear problems. His mother thought that in general there was much less mucus in his airways.

In sum, Guillermo became calmer, had fewer tantrums, and he himself said that he was less scared and having fewer nightmares, and therefore only sometimes got into his parents' bed. He is now also speaking much more clearly.

A runny nose is common in children of this age. Their physical proximity enables viruses to leave their 'native home' and allow new hosts the pleasure. However, if the runny nose turns into a real infection, then a visit first to the paediatrician and then to the pharmacy is usually on the agenda. Usually this means antibiotics, as it does here.

Susceptibility to infection
Leon, 4 years

Recorded by L.R., Shiatsu practitioner in Austria

For the past two months, according to his parents, Leon had been ill all the time. Every time he went to kindergarten, a day or two later he would have another bad cough, so bad that he had to stay at home again. Three weeks previously, on top of that, he had got inflammation of the middle ear. After taking antibiotics he would be free of problems for a couple of days, but then he would get another bad cough, with yellow catarrh streaming from his nose.

I offered to do a few Shōnishin treatments, and treated him from mid- April until mid-May – five sessions altogether. He enjoyed the treatments (basic treatment only) – so much that he even 'treated' his mother at home, she told me.

After the treatments Leon was no longer ill. His nose was less blocked and his cough had improved. It is true that now and again he had bit of a snuffle, but it no longer degenerated the way it had before the course of treatment.

In early June Leon came back because he was coughing again. I did another Shōnishin treatment, and up to now (four weeks later) the cough has not recurred.

Sometimes siblings have to be treated for the same problems – for example, sleep disturbance.

Sleep disturbance

Siblings – girl, 4 years; boy, 1½ years

Recorded by Dr D.S., doctor and spokesperson for training in acupuncture in Austria

Both siblings wake up four times, and are then lively during the night. The parents came for a consultation, I recommended Shōnishin.

Method used: basic treatment only.

Treatment 1: The children are relaxed, open, willing to cooperate.

Slept better the first night, woke up only twice.

Treatment 2: Looking forward to it.

Treatment 3: Sleep markedly improved, woke up once or twice.

Three weeks' break; got worse (waking up to three times).

Treatment 4: Sleep improved immediately.

Now coming only when required, about every two months, for one or two treatments.

A key effect of Shōnishin treatment is a calm, balanced state. Parents report this again and again, even if the child first came on account of entirely different complaints or symptoms. A good example of this is the next case history from a colleague in Vienna.

Behavioural problems

Lea, 5 years

Recorded by Dr L.R., doctor in Austria

Lea is my daughter. During the first three months she cried excessively. Her development was normal, but slow (hand–hand contact at 4 months, crawling at 10 months, walking on her own at 18 months).

Lea is an anxious girl with a strong will. She avoids being touched. In particular she will not let strangers touch her, and reacts (e.g. at the doctor's), with fits of rage, although she has never had an unpleasant experience there. She talks a lot and is very communicative, but takes a long time to make a connection with someone. If she doesn't get her own way, she immediately starts yelling. At night she grinds her teeth. She easily becomes car-sick.

Therapy: Altogether four times at weekly intervals, basic treatment and front family treatment (circuits) and yuan points.

Last week we went to the dentist. The three previous visits had been fruitless, she wouldn't open her mouth a single millimetre. This time she opened her mouth and let him take at least one X-ray. Now that's real progress!

12.4 Case studies – 6–13-year-olds

Diagnoses

- Multiple warts

- Primary enuresis

- Enuresis

- ADHD

- KISS syndrome

- Proprioceptive disorder

- Hyperventilation syndrome

- Sleep disturbance

On reaching school age, energetic development is temporarily complete, but not always! Increasingly, besides the yuan points, selected acupuncture points are included in the therapy plan for Shōnishin treatment. Whether these extra points are stimulated by means of vibration technique or by acupressure at home is decided on a case-by-case basis.

The following two examples provided by a colleague show how the mothers were involved in treating their sons by being shown particular acupuncture points to treat with acupressure. The first study concerns a tenacious case of warts.

Multiple warts

Gabriel, 6½ years

Recorded by Dr L.R., general practitioner in a hospital department for complementary medicine in Italy

Gabriel had lots of warts in his gluteal fold. The dermatologist recommended removing them under general anaesthetic, as there were so many that outpatient surgery would have been too much for the child. So, at his mother's request, Gabriel was cross-referred to our department.

Therapy: I treated Gabriel with Shōnishin four times at weekly intervals; just basic treatment for the first two sessions. After that I did the front circuit as well. In addition, I showed the mother points LI 4, Lu 7, SJ 5 and St 36, and advised her to apply acupressure on these points once a day.

One week after the first treatment the number of warts had decreased by half. After the third treatment only three warts were still visible, and a week later there was nothing to be seen.

Mother mentioned at the last session that Gabriel had been calmer since having therapy.

And here is the second example in which Shōnishin combined with acupressure was very successful.

Primary enuresis
Leonardo, 7 years

Recorded by Dr L.R., general practitioner in a hospital department for complementary medicine in Italy

Progression of treatment: Showed mother the point on the ulnar end of the distal palmar crease of the little fingers and on the lateral side of the end of the little toes near the corner of the nail. She was to massage these for ten days (approx. 30 seconds).

One-week interval, three cycles in all. In addition I treated Leonardo with Shōnishin six times at weekly intervals (basic treatment, reaction zone in the lumbar area, back *keiraku*).

After approximately 14 days he was dry almost every night. After five weeks he was completely dry.

As you can see, I like to combine my therapies with acupressure.

The issue of bedwetting is burdensome for everyone who has anything to do with it: in the first place, of course, for the affected child and parents, for which reason this problem is a constant subject of attention within the family. But this issue also concerns the Shōnishin acupuncturist and other therapists dealing with bedwetting, as it's such a hard nut to crack! The 'success quota' is not very high – in my practice it is around 30 per cent. The parents also need to be aware of this – so as not to raise false hopes, and also eliminate the pressure to succeed in one's own practice.

The example above and the one below show that bedwetting should not be seen as an absolutely hopeless problem – Shōnishin can still make a difference.

Enuresis

Lennart, nearly 7 years

Recorded by M.S., midwife in Germany

Lennart wets the bed up to twice a night. He has been going to school since the autumn and his bedwetting is very upsetting for him. I was his midwife when he was born. Two months ago he became a 'big brother' for the second time. His parents are separated and he has less contact with his father. I looked after his mother during labour, so his problem often came up in conversation.

He goes to bed at 8.00pm and his mother wakes him up at 11.00pm to go to the toilet. This he does almost in his sleep and often can't remember being woken up.

Lennart was very open to being treated and we had connected well when I was visiting his mother following delivery. He was allowed to decide whether he wished to be treated. Yes, he did, and after two treatments his mother told me that he would stand at the window waiting for me.

I did five treatments altogether: first, the basic treatment, and as meridian treatment the back family *keiraku*, which I also strengthened via its yuan points He 7, SI 4, Bl 64 and Ki 3. In addition, I tapped the kidney zone in the *hara* region (7x) and the reaction zone according to M. Tanioka on the back (7x). Whenever I was tapping on his front, Lennart couldn't help laughing a lot. Otherwise he enjoyed treatment – on a blanket in front of the stove. Following the first treatment he didn't wet the bed (twice), but he was still woken up at 11.00pm.

From the second treatment onwards I decided, apart from the treatment plan described above, to do front family meridian treatment as well (treating the circuit). I wanted to provide more support for his centre and reinforce his feeling of being taken care of (in spite of increased competition with siblings). The result was really impressive! He didn't wet the bed once, and appeared much more relaxed and happy. He was still woken up at 11.00pm to go to the toilet.

I did the third treatment in the same way as the second: basic treatment, front family circuit, back family *keiraku* and yuan points, kidney zone in the *hara* and reaction zone according to M. Tanioka. Again he stayed dry, except for one night, and was woken up at 11.00pm.

From the fourth treatment onwards he was not woken up, and didn't wet the bed!

Lennart wished for today's treatment as a 'booster' for everything to stay like this. He is very pleased and wrote me a little letter thanking me for my help. I was deeply touched. His mother is amazed at the great success of this simple, brief treatment and is making sure that method becomes more widely available.

Once they start school, children discover that they have to sit for far longer than they have so far been accustomed to do. For many children this can mean being unable to put up with sitting in class for so long. All too soon ideas of 'hyperactivity', 'attention deficit disorder', 'poor concentration' or 'ADHD' come up.

In the following example a colleague describes the case of a boy already branded with a diagnosis of ADHD.

ADHD

Christopher, 7½ years

Recorded by Dr S.F., general practitioner in private practice in Germany

After the paediatrician had diagnosed Christopher with ADHD and proposed Ritalin therapy to his mother, she sought an alternative way of treating the ADHD symptoms, as she had reservations about the medication.

Apart from a predisposition to dental caries, there was nothing significant in the previous medical history; in particular, birth and early development were normal. At the time of his first visit Christopher was in the preparatory class. Since leaving kindergarten, he was increasingly attracting attention because of his disruptive behaviour. But 'when he wanted to' he could also keep himself busy for an hour with his Playmobil. He also had huge problems getting to sleep (mother: 'He just won't settle down!'). His parents were particularly concerned about his verbal aggression towards them ('F**k you!') and the sudden fits of rage that he would have at the least provocation, especially if he didn't get his own way. If everything got too much for him, he tended to be sick.

On physical examination it was noted that he had rounded shoulders and overall hypotonic posture; he also had difficulty sitting still.

Three days after first contact I began treatment, which I did altogether eight times, in a weekly rhythm. The treatment (exclusively Shōnishin) lasted for approximately 8–10 minutes. Treatment consisted of two elements: basic treatment and specific treatment.

The specific treatment, in turn, consisted of three elements: 1) tapping treatment on the neck/shoulders area (*kanmushi* reaction zone according to Tanioka); 2) meridian treatment on the back family *keiraku* (motor restlessness with hypotonic body tone; inner restlessness with sleep disturbance); 3) vibration technique on the back *keiraku* yuan points.

Progression

First and second sessions: basic treatment, meridian treatment and back *keiraku* yuan points.

At the beginning of the third session his mother thought she could see a positive development in Christopher (less fidgety).

From the third session onwards: as above – additional tapping treatment.

At the fifth session Christopher's mother said that he had become much calmer. This state lasted until the eighth session, and so we agreed that I would see him again after an interval of eight weeks. At this next appointment Christopher's mother said that he could now concentrate for 30 minutes in lessons, and that he had had one violent tantrum. So we agreed that if he had any more tantrums we would do a few more Shōnishin treatments.

After the autumn holiday that followed (Christopher was now in the first year) he was brought back to see me, since he had become more fidgety since starting school again and kept having tantrums at home. Three more Shōnishin treatments (the same as in the third session) were done, in a weekly rhythm. At the third treatment his mother said that he was paying more attention, joining in more at school, and at home even consenting to do his homework.

Another appointment was made for six months later. Christopher's mother told me that he no longer had any sleep disturbances, rarely had tantrums, and was cooperating at school without any problems – and this without Ritalin or anything like it.

The next case study is also about ADHD. Luisa's case, from my own practice, shows that ADHD-like symptoms can mask other causes.

KISS syndrome

Luisa, 8 years

When I met Luisa she was 8 years old and in her third year at school. Owing to her restlessness and poor concentration she had been diagnosed with ADHD, and Ritalin therapy, urged by her class teacher, was planned.

Her mother, a single parent for the past two years, told me that she had noticed Luisa's restlessness and jumpiness while she was still at kindergarten. Now, last week at school, for example, she had simply stood up in the middle of a lesson and run around the room. When she had to sit down again, she picked up a pencil and tried to snap it. Because she couldn't, she drove it furiously into the table top until the point broke off.

Sitting still on a chair at all was very difficult for her; she would constantly slide back and forth or rock on the chair. And now her moving up into the next class was in jeopardy. Her mother told me how Luisa had already had three lots of treatment with different therapies: behavioural therapy, play therapy and learning therapy. 'As you can see, it's got us nowhere!' she concluded.

The first thing that struck me on examining Luisa was her asymmetrical head posture: her head was inclined slightly to the left, with restricted left rotation of the head (right rotation 85°, left rotation 70°), left shoulder lower than the right, scoliosis – not marked but still impossible to overlook (but not spotted in her pre-school medical examination!), pelvic tilt. The motor movement tests were unremarkable. For me, plenty of signs of KISS syndrome! My suspicions appeared to be confirmed by photos of Luisa in her first three months: in all of them, her head was rotated to the right.

And after further precise questioning I felt that my diagnosis stood on firm foundations: Luisa had cried a lot in the first three months, sleeping was 'a catastrophe'. Breastfeeding proved very difficult, especially at the right breast – she would 'lock on', but then would always instantly get worked up and start 'yelling at the breast'. She wouldn't lie on her tummy at all, and 'well, I had to do physiotherapy with her for three months!' She pulled herself along, never crawled, and could walk on her own at 18 months.

Then I examined her cervical spine. There was a blockage between the atlas and axis (segment C1/C2), which had obviously been there from birth. I treated the blockage with cranio-sacral therapy and chiropractic.

After that I did altogether six Shōnishin treatments (one a week). In the first three sessions I treated the front family, to support the external as well as the internal centre, which she had not been able to form in infancy owing to the asymmetry. The fourth to sixth sessions I devoted to the back family, because in my view what lay behind Luisa's restlessness was not ADHD but a weak back. Sitting for a long time makes a weak back hurt, distracting from what is actually happening (e.g. classwork). The backache can be tolerated only by keeping moving – it's easy to see that then there isn't enough energy left over to concentrate on anything.

As Luisa's problems, or the causes of her problems, had been there from birth, the three families couldn't develop freely. That is also the reason I treated her on the circuit level of the family, rather than the level of the *keiraku* or the five phases.

It cannot be said that Luisa developed into a calm child. Even so – medicinal therapy was now redundant. Luisa is now 11 years old; she is known as a very vivacious girl with lots of ideas and a liking for untidiness. At school she is not seen as a high flier, but her school achievements are still around the 'good average' mark.

Shōnishin can serve as the cornerstone of a therapy plan for proprioceptive problems; through treatment techniques like stroking or tapping, it addresses different perceptual systems (e.g. the tactile and proprioceptive systems).

Proprioceptive disorder
Tim, 10 years

Recorded by Dr A.R., doctor in Austria

Tim has a 4-year-old sister, Mum is pregnant with her third child, and the family is currently living in a very cramped two-room apartment. Tim is about to enter his first year at grammar school.

Case history: Normal pregnancy, spontaneous birth, but with vacuum extractor support during protracted labour. According to Mum, it was already noticeable at birth that he was rather 'lazy'. All in all he was late at every stage of development, and didn't crawl at all. First attempts at walking at 13 months; only retroactively, at age 2 and after a lot of motivational work, did he learn to crawl.

Since the age of 1 Tim has 'moved' six times (place of residence as well as social settings like kindergarten and school), as Mum was still studying at the time he was born. Dad is Dutch and the children are being brought up bilingual, but it is clear that the main language at home is German.

To begin with, Tim really liked having a sister, but only up to the time when she began moving around independently. After that there were big problems between the siblings for almost two years, partly because Tim's sister was already able to do things that he hadn't yet learnt to do.

Mum describes Tim as a 'little Buddha' as a baby and toddler, and says that a photo of him in his high chair at the dining table with some food in his hand is very characteristic. At the same time she says she has the feeling that Tim often has no sense of himself: he's always getting new scratches, bruises, wounds, and if he forgets to brake and rides his bike into a wall there seems to be no learning effect and he does it twice more. Often he himself doesn't seem to notice his injuries; if you ask him about them he's very surprised and doesn't know where it happened this time.

As Mum herself is a doctor and uses alternative medicine, she has already tried out lots of different therapies on Tim (or taken him to alternative therapists for treatment): physiotherapy, occupational therapy, acupuncture…

Tim can read and write well (to begin with, fine motor skills were difficult, but now he enjoys it very much), has a good imagination and endless patience (he can stick at things for a long time). He has very high comprehension skills (Mum: 'bone idle and highly gifted'), and a very good vocabulary (in conversation with me he uses words like 'avoiding conflict' and 'complex' in the appropriate context).

Treatment: Basic treatment plus front family circuit treatment, plus emphasis on the centre (tapping the spleen area around the navel), plus front family yuan. Three treatments up to now.

My opinion: Mum says that when she does acupuncture on Tim herself, she emphasises the centre above all, so I also decided on front family treatment for the obvious lack of coordination, lack of sensitivity to pain and marked early difficulties with reading and writing. Mum says she thinks he has been a little calmer over the last few days.

Nevertheless, next time I would begin to treat the back family circuit, since for me, now that I know Tim a bit better, the main issues in the case history seem to be 'not sensing himself' (proprioceptive system) and missing out crawling. At the first treatment Tim also asked for deeper pressure; at the second treatment, during which I stayed with gentler pressure rather than do as he had asked, he did show a better response.

All in all I believe that Tim needs 'stronger backing', especially now that the third child is on the way. His parents are already treating him as very grown up; he helps a lot at home, is very independent, has quite sophisticated discussions with me during treatment, but in all this sometimes gives the appearance of simply being rather lost and out of his depth. Oddly enough, I would have described his mum (a colleague of mine) in just the same way as she describes her son – 'He has no sense of himself!' – I find her just like that in the way she deals with patients and colleagues, and in certain situations.

In the next example a symptom – in this case, breathing difficulty – is making its first appearance in a 10-year-old boy. The death of his grandfather had thrown him off centre.

Hyperventilation syndrome

Boy, 10 years

Recorded by A.H., complementary therapist in Germany

The boy is brought to see me by his father because of sporadic shortness of breath. He has already had a medical examination, with negative results.

He had been experiencing difficulty breathing for approximately two weeks. It happened quite suddenly, out of the blue, sometimes after a meal – altogether about 12 times up to now. Then the child would also have numbness in his hands and feet.

In conversation it turned out that his grandfather had died not long before, and it was weighing heavily on the boy. He seemed introverted and kept himself to himself.

To get an idea of how bad it was, I asked him to rate it on a scale of 1 to 10 – with 1 being 'not much' and 10 being 'a lot'.

He rated the breathing problem as '5–6'.

Big, deep sadness was '8'.

THERAPY

Basic treatment, meridian treatment of two phases: wood (spleen–stomach) and metal (lung–large intestine) and their yuan points.

After the treatment we had a good, enriching conversation.

One week later: The boy rates the breathing difficulty '3–4', it's occurring less frequently and is noticeably less severe, the sadness he feels is '4'.

Treatment as on the first occasion.

One week later: His general condition appears good; he seems very open and talks about football. He says the breathing trouble has gone ('0'); he misses his grandfather, of course, but now he can once again feel happy, and enjoy life too.

Treatment for the last time, as before.

I discharged the boy, symptom-free. I know the family through the football team, and heard that there was no recurrence of the breathing problem.

The following example from my own practice shows how important it is to pay attention to the underlying cause of a given problem, and the time of its first appearance.

Sleep disturbance

Larissa, 13 years

Larissa had never had 'real problems', her mother told me on their first visit. Even the pregnancy had been problem-free. Nothing untoward in the spontaneous delivery. The first time she rolled from her back onto her tummy was at five months, proper crawling at eight months, and walking on her own at 13 months. At kindergarten Larissa was very popular with the teachers and the children because of her friendliness and love of being with others. She and her best friend were 'one heart and soul', her mother said.

The problem started when she entered the fifth year [at school]: Larissa could no longer sleep through the night. Since then, night after night, she had been waking up to three times, and then couldn't get back to sleep for ages. And this had now been going on for four years. The whole family was very unhappy about it.

When Larissa was 11 her mother took her to see a paediatrician because of the increasing strain she was under. He was of the opinion that the move to grammar school and corresponding pressure to achieve had been too much for Larissa, and recommended transferring to the comprehensive school. But seeing that Larissa was not having any problems, either with the school in general, or with her academic performance specifically, her parents did not follow the paediatrician's advice.

The distress kept getting worse, as she was unable to sleep through, even for a single night. In contrast to the way it had been at the onset of the sleep disturbance when she was 10, now, at 12, she would lie awake, sometimes for hours, with her head full of thoughts. So she and her mother went to see a child psychologist. Because she was entering puberty (she had not yet begun to menstruate) he concluded that she was just discovering her sexuality, and that that was the reason for her 'hefty awake phases'. Larissa did not go back to the child psychologist.

On the advice of a friend of her mother's, the next port of call was the osteopath. He examined Larissa and found that the fascia of her liver was too tense. He eased the tension, and Larissa still couldn't sleep through the night. Then he said that the reason must be disturbance of the cranio-sacral rhythm. But even after the rhythm had been restored, everything was still the same as before.

Three months before Larissa visited my practice the paediatrician prescribed 'a mild sedative' for her. It enabled her to sleep through the night – however, the result was that she woke up in the morning feeling 'wrung out', as if she had had anything but a good night's sleep. After a six-week 'trial period' she herself stopped taking the medication. For the last five weeks she had been going to a complementary therapist, who during that time had done ten sessions of needle acupuncture with her. I asked to see the acupuncture points: I could make out Du 20, Ki 3 and He 7. Apart from the fact that she had found some of the needling very painful, it had had no effect. So much for her previous history.

After hearing this tale of woe I asked Larissa whether anything else had happened during this time, apart from the move to grammar school. Yes, they had moved house. In reply to my question about what it had been like for her, she said that she had cried for several days because she had been separated from her friends, especially her best friend. She said that at the time she had frequently also had bad tummy ache.

With that, the cause was clear to me: Larissa had been uprooted by moving house. The treatment had to begin from there!

Treatment strategy: Restore the feeling of being at home in herself.

Procedure: Basic treatment, meridian treatment of the earth phase, yuan points of spleen and stomach meridians, periumbilical tapping treatment, permanent needle (0.6mm) at Ren 12.

We agreed on six sessions; after four sessions we broke off treatment because since the third session she had not once woken up at night. She came back four weeks later: there had been no more sleep problems.

12.5 Case studies – Adults

Diagnoses

- Whiplash injury
- Headache with vertigo
- Breast cancer
- Fibromyalgia
- Multimorbidity

Shōnishin has an important role to play in the treatment of adults. Besides being commonly used in cases of needle phobia, Shōnishin can be a valuable adjunct to other methods of treatment (complementary or mainstream), as the following case studies show.

The combination of Shōnishin with acupuncture, chiropractic or cranio-sacral therapy has been proven many times in treatment of the head, neck and shoulders. Here is a report from an outpatient pain clinic.

Whiplash injury

Bettina M., 31 years

> Recorded by Dr I.W., consultant in anaesthesia and intensive care in Austria
>
> Female patient suffered a whiplash injury in a road accident approximately seven months ago. (Another car drove into her sideways from the rear.) In the first days after the accident: increasing pain and restricted movement, also formication [a tingling sensation under the skin] at C7.
>
> MRI (one week after the accident): Loss of cervical lordosis, otherwise no significant findings, with no sign of oedema in the medullary canal or soft tissue.
>
> Start physiotherapy and manual therapy. No lasting improvement after two cycles, only the formication has improved. The patient is still suffering from severe tensions in her neck and frequent headaches emanating from the neck, worsening when working at a computer. Her family doctor has now referred her for acupuncture.
>
> 27.7.2012: Start acupuncture (Bl 2, 10, 23, 60, Ki 3, Gb 20, LI 4, Pc 6).
>
> In addition, Shōnishin: basic treatment, with head and neck treatment, tapping technique on shoulder area.

The patient finds the treatment very pleasant, feels very relaxed and 'easier in my head'.

06.08.2012: Relaxed feeling lasted for approximately three days (longer than with everything else up to now).

Repeated the programme of acupuncture and Shōnishin. Again, the patient has a sense of wellbeing.

Then a break, as the patient is away on holiday. Since then, no further contact.

The patient in the following case was also successfully treated with Shōnishin combined with chiropractic.

Headache with vertigo
Teacher, 59 years

Recorded by P.E., complementary therapist in Germany

For eight years now Mrs G. has been coming to see me for headaches, which respond well to treatment with APM [Penzel Acupuncture Massage].

Two months ago she requested an urgent appointment. She was complaining of unpleasant rotatory and positional vertigo. As I didn't have enough time to do APM, I suggested doing three Shōnishin treatments.

Visual observation: Stressed, muscular hypertonus of the entire shoulder girdle, panic in her eyes.

Palpation: Atlas blocked on the left side; restricted rotation of the spinal column both sides; sacro-iliac joints blocked on right and left side; in the heart area of the *hara,* tender when touched; overall raised muscle tone.

Patient's experience: Afraid to lie down, massive sleep disturbance, no longer feels centred, anxious.

Treatment 1: Basic treatment, released the sacro-iliac blockage.

Treatment 2: Next day, much calmer, still has vertigo, eyes no longer so panicky.

Basic treatment, front family circuit treatment (incl. yuan points), tapping treatment on neck/shoulder area.

Treatment 3: Next day, no more vertigo at night, spinal column noticeably more mobile.

Treatment same as the day before, plus Shōnishin treatment on a scar on the head.

Treatment 4: Five days later, Mrs G. feels relaxed, no vertigo at night, calmer, still dizzy during the day if stressed.

Basic treatment, front family circuit treatment (incl. yuan points), again released the sacro-iliac blockage and showed exercises to be done at home.

Treatment 5: Stable condition, just basic treatment.

Treatment 6: Stable condition, just basic treatment.

For a patient with a serious and life-changing diagnosis, it is especially important to ease the load of a severe illness. For example, in treatment for cancer Shōnishin has been shown to be of value as an additional support for conventional therapy, in order to bring about – even if only temporarily – an improvement in their general condition.

Breast cancer

Mrs X, 64 years

Recorded by C.P., Shiatsu practitioner in Austria

Mrs X has been coming to me since 2010 on the recommendation of a complementary practitioner, mainly for Shiatsu treatment. She is of medium height, very slim, has very upright posture, appears very agile and active for her age, and has an infectious smile. Mrs X is married, has a grown-up daughter and loves exercise.

DIAGNOSES

Condition after operation: Solid carcinoma of the left breast with lumpectomy and 54 irradiations at 49.

Condition after operation: Solid carcinoma of the right breast with ablation without radiotherapy or chemotherapy at 60.

Breast reconstruction of the right breast from *M. latissimus dorsi* (at 61), with chronic pain in the scar on her back.

Chronic constipation.

SHŌNISHIN TREATMENT

In 2011 a lymph node in the right axilla, which was under surveillance, degenerated and later turned out to be encapsulated tissue from the right breast carcinoma. The node was surgically completely removed and there were no affected lymph nodes in the surrounding tissues. Nevertheless she had to have chemotherapy and adjuvant radiotherapy.

During the chemotherapy I switched treatment from Shiatsu to Shōnishin, as in my experience Shiatsu treatment can often be too much information for the body in such extreme situations. At the start of chemotherapy she was doing well enough under the circumstances, suffering not until after the third cycle from nausea, dry mouth, loss of appetite and constipation. It was at this stage that I changed the treatment to Shōnishin.

The basic treatment was always used. Some areas and additional points proved especially useful:

Vomiting/nausea:

> Tapping in the area of the reaction zone according to M. Tanioka
>
> Stroking around the navel
>
> Additional points such as Ren 12, St 25, Pc 6 and Pc 10, also Sp 4.

Constipation:

> Tapping from Bl 20 to Bl 25
>
> Stroking around the navel
>
> Additional points such as St 25, LI 4, Sp 6, St 36, Gb 34.

I always incorporated the points and additional areas into the basic treatment. Since at this time Mrs X was not comfortable lying on her front, I worked with her lying on her back in a slightly raised position, and on her side with a support cushion. The treatment, adjusted to fit in with the chemotherapy cycles, was always done on the second day after the drug infusion. This gave better control of nausea, appetite returned more quickly and the intestine was kept active. Mrs X always enjoyed the treatments very much, as they gave her the feeling of getting over the worst days better.

During the radiotherapy cycles I incorporated more Shiatsu, but still treated the special points and areas with the Shōnishin instrument, as Mrs X responded to it so well.

SUMMARY

Shōnishin during treatment for cancer has the advantage of being brief, precise and very effective. If the client feels unwell it is possible to have a break or change position, and treatment can also be done with the patient sitting. The treatment time can easily be adapted to the patient's current state of health. Shōnishin is ideal for soothing acute symptoms, but in my experience subsequent Shiatsu therapy is helpful for maintaining improvement if there are chronic problems.

The power of gentleness can be seen in the next example, in which conventional medical treatments – both complementary and mainstream – were unsuccessful. The therapeutic breakthrough came with Shōnishin.

Fibromyalgia
Woman, 61 years

> Recorded by Professor R.W., MD, Department of General Paediatrics and Adolescent Medicine, Division of Neonatology in Austria
>
> Female patient, 61 years old, eight months' pain and feeling of weakness in the extremities, suspected fibromyalgia (diagnosed in March 2012).
>
> Many attempts to treat by diet/elimination of fructose/ear acupuncture (patient has needle phobia)/Schüssler salts, with different doctors. Currently on a combination of three analgesics. Severe weight loss of 10kg in two months because of intolerable pain, restricted mobility – no longer able to drive.
>
> I did a basic treatment with the patient, of the strength that would be used for a 10–12-year-old child, as she reacts with extreme sensitivity. There was approximately 30 per cent improvement after the first treatment. After the third treatment 50 per cent, and now, after the fifth treatment, she has been completely pain-free for 6 weeks continuously.

Being able to do something good for a person can mean a great deal. Older patients all too rarely have the experience of good things happening to them – especially when they have to have therapeutic treatment. They find therapy disagreeable, sometimes painful too, and taking medicine doesn't necessarily bring about an improvement in their health.

But what old people suffer from especially is lack of caring attention. Conventional medicine has neither time nor place for it. Shōnishin can fill this gap, thanks to the distinctive nature of the attention that it offers – and the therapy feels pleasant too. This is a great help in getting things moving.

The next case looks at one particular aspect of treatment in older people – the skin. In old people it is thin, easily damaged and sometimes parchment-like. Many old people are on anticoagulant medication, because of which any kind of injury (e.g. bursting of a blood vessel because of excessive pressure) is to be avoided. Consequently, the stroking technique is done not at the normal strength for adults, but as for 2–3-year-olds, or in many cases even younger children.

Multimorbidity (following heart attack, severe PAOD [peripheral arterial occlusive disease], pain in joints and throughout the spine, sleep disturbance)

Woman, 86 years

Recorded by Dr C.S., paediatrician in Austria

The patient is my grandma. She has always been a very active person, accustomed to being there for everybody and taking care of everything. Mentally she is in tip-top condition, but because of her pain and underlying illness she can no longer do as much as she would like to and is terribly unhappy about that. Pain medication helps only a little, and after every infusion she has an enormous haematoma.

Because of her thin and sensitive skin I thought of gentle Shōnishin, so as to cause the least possible irritation. I just wanted to do her good; it was not my intention to cure any of her illnesses.

I visited her five times and every time did just the basic treatment. Every time following treatment she slept much better and was relaxed. She felt better generally. That alone was success for both of us.

Now every time we meet she wants me to give her a treatment, and it makes her happy.

Feedback

Shōnishin is a valuable extension of my paediatric work. Every day I have occasion to use it, and patients, parents and I myself can see the results of this gentle acupuncture... Up to now no method I have learnt has been so successful in practice – thank you so much. From excessive crying to bedwetting and even ADHD, I have had unexpected success where all else had failed – could be chance, but it seems to happen too often for that. Super!

(Dr Förster, paediatrician, Salzburg)

I am thrilled with your course and the opportunity to learn this technique from you.

(Professor R. Weitzdoerfer, Department of General Paediatrics and Adolescent Medicine, Division of Neonatology, Medical University of Vienna)

I have had great fun with Shōnishin over the last few weeks. I am impressed by the effect of this method. In general I have had fantastic results, often with just the basic treatment.

(Dr J. Rojas-Stütz, paediatrician, Mexico City)

I keep being 'bowled over' by this method. Already five children have been symptom-free after four to eight sessions. Incredible! And their poor mothers had been so desperate. Just today I had another message in my Combox from one of the mothers, thanking me a thousand times for the Shōnishin treatments. Her little girl had been unable to sleep properly for three years after suffering a trauma. Now she sleeps like an angel every night.

(Sabine Bannwart, Shiatsu practitioner, Zürich)

Maya was brought to the practice at the age of 4 months with the following diagnosis: postural asymmetry, skewed to the right, following a forceps delivery. Her parents said that Maya was a very restless child, crying at night and during the day.

On examining her I found high-degree functional disorder of the suboccipital joints on the right, and very tense paravertebral and suboccipital musculature.

I know that children with such tense muscles cry a lot during treatment with manual therapy. Therefore I prepared Maya with Shōnishin beforehand and let her rest for 30 minutes. Then when I treated her, she scarcely cried during treatment. After the treatment she settled down very quickly and smiled at me. Since then I have almost always treated children in this way: first Shōnishin, then manual therapy. The children react much more calmly to my treatment and there are hardly any vegetative reactions (pallor, breaking out in a sweat, etc.).

(Dr Svetlana Iliaeva, Consultant in Physical Medicine, Cologne)

Lennart is very happy and wrote me a little letter thanking me for my help. I was deeply moved. His mother is amazed at this brief, simple treatment and the great success it has had, and is eager to spread the word about the method. I am grateful to Lennart for being my cheerful and expectant 'guinea-pig' (*Author's note*: the midwife was training for the Certificate in Shōnishin), and I can say how glad I am to have learned this form of therapy.

(Marion Stöber, midwife)

Bibliography

Baumann, T. *Atlas der Entwicklungsdiagnostik.* Thieme, Stuttgart 2007

Bein-Wierzbinski, W. *Das PäPKi®-Konzept Manuelle Med*, 2011, 49, p. 154

Behrends, J.C. 'Sinnesphysiologie: Funktionsprinzipien und somatoviszerable Sensibilität.' In *Duale Reihe Physiologie*, Thieme, Stuttgart 2010, p. 604

Biedermann, H. *Kopfgelenk-induzierte Symmetriestörungen bei Kleinkindern.* der kinderarzt 1991, 22, pp. 1475–1482

Biedermann, H. 'KISS-Kinder.' In T. Harms (ed.) *Auf die Welt gekommen.* Ulrich Leutner Verlag, Berlin 2000

Birch, S. *Shonishin: Japanese Pediatric Acupuncture.* Thieme, Stuttgart 2011

Buchmann, J., Bülow, B. *Funktionelle Kopfgelenksstörung im Zusammenhang mit Lagereaktionen und Tonusasymmetrie.* Manuelle Med, 1983, 21, pp. 59–62

Coenen, W. *Bewegungsstörungen im Säuglingsalter.* Manuelle Med, 2011, 49, p. 173

Cranenburgh, B. van. *Segmentale Phänomene.* Kiener, München 2012

Deutzmann, R. 'Hormonelle Regulation.' In *Duale Reihe Physiologie*, Thieme 2010

Ekiken, K. *Regeln zur Lebenspflege (Yōjōkun).* Iudicium Verlag, München 2010

Flaws, B. *Chinesische Heilkunde für Kinder.* Joy Verlag 2007, p.153

Gleditsch, J. *MAPS, MikroAkuPunktSysteme: Grundlagen und Praxis der somatotopischen Therapie.* Hippokrates, Stuttgart 2002

Helmer, R. *Treating Pediatric Bed-wetting with Acupuncture & Chinese Medicine.* Blue Poppy Press 2006

Herold, R. *Zur Sozialisation des Kindes im Japan der Tokugawa- und Meiji-Zeit.* OAG aktuell 1993, p. 60

Kalbantner-Wernicke, K. *Shiatsu für Babys und Kleinkinder. Energetische Entwicklung, Förderung und Behandlung.* Elsevier 2010

Kalbantner-Wernicke, K., Wernicke, T. *Baby-Shiatsu – eine energetische Ergänzung zur osteopathischen Behandlung.* Osteopathische Medizin, 2010, pp. 10–13

Kappstein, S. *Akupressur bei Kindern.* Hippokrates-Verlag, Stuttgart 1982

Kuklinski, B. *Das HWS-Trauma.* AURUM-Verlag 2007

Larre C., Rochat de la Vallee, E. *Chinese Medicine from the Classics: 'the heart in lingshu chapter 8'.* Monkey Press 1991

Loebell, P. In *Erziehungskunst*, 2012, 1, S.59

Mackenzie, J. *Krankheitszeichen und ihre Auslegung.* Leipzig, Kabitsch 1921

Manaka, Y. *Manakas Quantensprung.* ML Verlag, Uelzen 2004

Nagano. 'Praxis Shōnishin.' In Ozaki Tomofumi, Yamaguchi Hajime, Yoneyama Sakae (eds) *Jissen shōnihari-hō – kodomo no sukoyakana seichō e no apurōchi*. Ishiyaku Shuppan, Tōkyō 2012

Rotermund, H.O. *Säcke der Weisheit und Meere des Wissens. Alte japanische Hausbücher – Ein kulturgeschichtliches Lesebuch*. Iudicium Verlag, München 2010

Römer, A. *Akupunktur für Hebammen, Geburtshelfer und Gynäkologen*. Hippokrates Verlag, Stuttgart 2008

Sacher, R. 'Geburtstrauma und (Hals-)Wirbelsäule.' In Biedermann (ed.) *Manuelle Therapie bei Kindern*. Elsevier 2006

Scott, J., Barlow, T. *Akupunktur in der Behandlung von Kindern*. Verlag für Ganzheitliche Medizin Dr. Erich Wühr, 2003, p. 288

Schellenberg, I. Schellenberg, C., Reiche, D., Blanck, N. *Kinderkrankheiten von A–Z. Das Handbuch*. Haug 2009

Schleip, R. *Die Bedeutung der Faszien in der manuellen Therapie*. Dt Ztschr f Osteop, 2004, 1, S.13

Schneider, F. (ed.) *Klinikmanual Psychiatrie, Psychosomatik und Psychotherapie*. Springer, Heidelberg 2008

Seifert, I. *Kopfgelenksblockierungen bei Neugeborenen. Rehabilitacia (Suppl)*. 1975, 10/11, 53–56

Shou-chuan ,W., Mulin Qiao-Wong, J., Xia, Z. *Pediatrics in Chinese Medicine*. People's Medical Publishing House, 2012

Uvnäs-Moberg, K., Arn, I., Magnusson, D. *The psychobiology of emotion: the role of the oxytocinergic system*. Int J Behav Med, 2005, 12, 59–65

Tanioka, M. *Taishiryu-Shōnishin ('Shōnishin nach der Daishi-Schule')*. Verlag Rikuzensha, 2005

Waldeyer, *Anatomie des Menschen, 17*. Auflage, Berlin 2003, p. 99

Wancura-Kampik, I. *Segment-Anatomie*. Elsevier, München 2009

Wernicke, T. *Shōnishin – japanische Kinderakupunktur*. Elsevier, München 2009

Wernicke, T., Kalbantner-Wernicke, K. *Kinderakupunktur mit der entwicklungsphysiologisch orientierten Shōnishin-Methode*. Dt Ztschr f Akup, 2009, 49, 2, pp. 18–24

Yoneyama, H., Mori, H. *The Method of Shoni-shin*. Ido no Nippon sha 1964

Ziegler, M., Wollwerth, R., Papousek, M. 'Exzessives Schreien im frühen Säuglingsalter.' In M. Papousek, M. Schieche, H. Wurmser (eds) *Regulationsstörungen der frühen Kindheit*. Verlag Hans Huber, 2004

Index